THE COMPLETE GUIDE TO
HEALING ARTHRITIS

**Books in the Healthy Home Library Series
from St. Martin's Paperbacks**

A Woman's Guide to Vitamins, Herbs and Supplements
by Deborah Mitchell

The Complete Book of Nutritional Healing
by Deborah Mitchell

The Complete Guide to Living Well with Diabetes
by Winifred Conkling

*The Concise Encyclopedia of Women's Sexual
and Reproductive Health*
by Deborah Mitchell

25 Medical Tests Your Doctor Should Tell You About...
by Deborah Mitchell

52 Foods and Supplements for a Healthy Heart
by Deborah Mitchell

How to Live Well With Early Alzheimer's
by Deborah Mitchell

The Anti-Cancer Food and Supplement Guide
by Debora Yost

The Family Guide to Vitamins, Herbs, and Supplements
by Deborah Mitchell

The Complete Guide to Lowering Your Cholesterol
by Mary Mihaly

The Complete Guide to Healing Fibromyalgia
by Deborah Mitchell

The Complete Guide to Healing Arthritis
by Deborah Mitchell

THE COMPLETE GUIDE TO HEALING ARTHRITIS

Deborah Mitchell

A Lynn Sonberg Book

St. Martin's Paperbacks

THE COMPLETE GUIDE TO HEALING ARTHRITIS

Copyright © 2011 by Lynn Sonberg Book Associates.

All rights reserved.

For information address St. Martin's Press, 175 Fifth Avenue, New York, NY 10010.

EAN: 978-0-312-53416-5

Printed in the United States of America

St. Martin's Paperbacks edition / April 2011

St. Martin's Paperbacks are published by St. Martin's Press, 175 Fifth Avenue, New York, NY 10010.

10   9   8   7   6   5   4   3   2

CONTENTS

THE COMPLETE GUIDE TO
HEALING ARTHRITIS

INTRODUCTION

"I've got a touch of arthritis."

"It's just my arthritic knee acting up."

"I've got arthritis in my [fill in the blank]."

These are phrases you hear often, and that's no surprise when you consider that an estimated 47 million adults in America live with some form of arthritis and another nearly three hundred thousand young people have a type of the disease as well. By 2030, it is projected that there will be 67 million Americans living with some form of the syndrome.

When I talk about arthritis in this book, I am focusing primarily on the most common type of the disease, the one that most people are referring to when they talk about arthritis and the one that affects approximately 27 million Americans: osteoarthritis.

However, I also devote a great deal of discussion to two "other" forms of arthritis—rheumatoid arthritis and gout. These two forms of arthritis affect fewer individuals—an estimated 3.1 million Americans have rheumatoid arthritis and about 3 million have gout—yet they have a significant impact on the lives of the people who have developed these conditions. Both forms of arthritis can be debilitating, especially rheumatoid arthritis, which is one of the most serious and damaging forms of arthritis. Thus this book is about how to face, manage, and live life to the fullest with osteoarthritis, rheumatoid arthritis, and gout.

I also take a brief but informative look at about a dozen other types of arthritis and arthritis-related conditions. While they are much less common than osteoarthritis, it is good to have a basic understanding of these types of arthritis, as it is not uncommon for people who have osteoarthritis to have another type of arthritis as well and the combination can make both diagnosis and treatment a challenge.

HOW TO USE THIS BOOK

Arthritis is a condition that has garnered a lot of research, and in this volume I present the latest findings and information in two different categories. In part 1 I lay the groundwork for a basic understanding of osteoarthritis, rheumatoid arthritis, and gout and the impact they can have on your health and lifestyle. I briefly explore an additional ten types of arthritis that are somewhat less common but that may develop along with any of the three main types of arthritis that I focus on in this book. Part 1 also covers how to find the most appropriate health-care providers to work with you and offers a comprehensive look at how doctors make a diagnosis of arthritis. Throughout the chapters in part 1 I refer you to sections in part 2 for treatment options and tips and guidelines on how to face the daily challenges that having arthritis can bring.

In part 2 I delve into how to live with arthritis on a daily basis. This includes information on a wealth of treatment choices, ranging from exercise and physical therapy to nutritional and other natural supplements, alternative/complementary body and mind therapies, conventional medications, medical procedures and surgeries, and assistive devices. Much has been and continues to evolve in these areas, and I provide the most up-to-date information available. I also explore where you can find support in this fast-growing technological age, the many different ideas about diet and which foods are best—and worst—for arthritis, and how to cope with some everyday challenges associated with having arthritis, such as sexual problems, managing housework, how to recover after surgery for arthritis, ways to deal with fatigue, and much more.

Arthritis may be a part of your life, but it need not define who you are. I hope you will read through this book and find new ways to live with arthritis, ideas that will motivate you to talk to your health-care provider about new treatments or activities and overall improve your quality of life. Please feel free to share what you read and learn with your family, friends, and others who may have arthritis.

PART I

Arthritis 101

CHAPTER ONE

Arthritis: An Introduction

Perhaps you shrugged it off the first few times you experienced it: an uncomfortable feeling in your knee, the lingering pain in your lower back when you got up in the morning, the slight change in flexibility in your hands. Maybe you have begun needing help opening jars. The stairs may be a bit more painful to climb. You hear a grating or popping sound in your lower back when you move a certain way. And the most unsettling part for you is that these symptoms are not going away. That's when it may have occurred to you: "I wonder if it's arthritis?"

You are part of a large and growing population of people of all ages who has what is generally and commonly referred to as arthritis. It is a big disease: it affects tens of millions of people, has the ability to impact every aspect of their lives, is the subject of much continuing research being conducted into its many facets, and is associated with an impressive number of conventional and alternative treatments and management options. Much has been written about it in scientific literature, on the Internet, and in books and magazines.

This chapter is an introduction to the concept of arthritis and specifically the most common type of the disease:

osteoarthritis. I bring together the most relevant, up-to-date information available on osteoarthritis with the hope of helping you better manage, live with, and rise above the challenges posed by this most common of all types of arthritis.

Let's get started.

WHAT IS THIS THING CALLED ARTHRITIS?

"Arthritis" literally means "joint inflammation." Even though this describes a symptom or sign rather than a specific diagnosis, most people use the term "arthritis" to refer to any condition that affects the joints.

The word "arthritis" is tossed around generically, but in reality the term describes not a single disease but rather more than one hundred different yet somewhat similar conditions that affect the joints, tendons, and muscles. Some types of arthritis also impact the skin and other organs. Of the more than one hundred different types of arthritis, only a handful are considered to be common and one alone accounts for about 60 percent of all cases of arthritis: osteoarthritis.

When most people talk about arthritis, they are usually referring to osteoarthritis. For the 3.1 million Americans who have the "other" arthritis, the term "rheumatoid arthritis" is what comes to mind. A third type of arthritis that often does not get the respect it deserves is gout, which affects more than 3 million people. All together, these three types of arthritis directly impact the lives of an estimated 33 million people, leaving the remaining 14 million individuals affected by any of the 100-plus types of arthritis that remain.

MYTHS ABOUT ARTHRITIS

Even though arthritis has been around for millennia, there are still many misconceptions and misunderstandings about what it is and what it is not. So here are a few of the more common myths and the truth:

- **Arthritis is just a name for aches and pains that affect older people.** At the risk of repeating myself, I emphasize that arthritis can affect people of any age, not just older people, and it can involve much more than aches and pains. If you are experiencing any of the signs and symptoms mentioned in this chapter or in chapter 2, you should see a health-care professional to get a diagnosis so you can start a plan of treatment and avoid as much disruption to your life as possible. Chapter 4 outlines how your doctor may diagnose arthritis.

- **Arthritis isn't that serious.** While we don't want to be alarmist, arthritis *is* a serious condition: it affects about one-third of adults and nearly three hundred thousand children in the United States. About one-third of people age 18 to 64 who have arthritis have arthritis-attributable work limitations. According to the 2005 Survey of Income and Program Participation, arthritis and other rheumatic conditions have been and continue to be the most common cause of disability in the United States. The latest figure for the total costs associated with arthritis and other rheumatic conditions in the United States was $128 billion in 2003, up from $86.2 billion in 1997.

- **There's no cure, so there's not much you can do about arthritis.** The absence of a cure definitely does not mean you can't achieve significant improvement in symptoms using exercise and body therapies, medications, natural remedies, and medical procedures. One of the most exciting things about arthritis today is that patients are learning that they can play a significant role in their own disease management by taking advantage of conventional and alternative therapy options and networking avenues. New research findings are released regularly on innovative ways to prevent and treat many different types of arthritis. In this book I explore treatment ideas in several different categories.

OSTEOARTHRITIS

Osteoarthritis is not only the most common type of arthritis and the one with the most name recognition; it is also the type that will affect one in two people during their lifetime. If you have ever suffered a knee injury, your risk for knee osteoarthritis rises to 57 percent. Are you obese? Now your risk for knee osteoarthritis has just climbed to 60 percent.

The Centers for Disease Control estimate there are 27 million adults who have osteoarthritis, also known as degenerative joint disease, but that just represents doctor-diagnosed cases. Millions of people are likely living with undiagnosed osteoarthritis, individuals who have chosen not to seek medical care because they feel they do not need it or that they can take care of their symptoms themselves or they may not have health insurance. Perhaps you are among the 27 million or the yet-undiagnosed millions, or maybe you have a loved one with the disease. In any case, here's the story on osteoarthritis.

What Does Osteoarthritis Look Like?

Imagine you are looking at the ends of the bones that form a joint. The two ends are cushioned by cartilage, like a piece of firm elastic or rubber that allows the joint to move smoothly and efficiently. Now picture the rubbery cartilage deteriorating, breaking away bit by bit, which allows the bone ends to rub against each other. Tiny pieces of bone or cartilage break off and float in the space between the bones and around the joint, causing irritation and pain.

The rubbing bones and cartilage can cause other changes, including the development of bony growths called spurs that can cause additional irritation. When the shape of the joint is altered, it can no longer function smoothly. The lining of the joint, called the synovium, becomes inflamed and causes proteins called cytokines to appear and damage the cartilage even further. The overall result is pain, stiffness, reduced function, and limited mobility: you have osteoarthritis.

Osteoarthritis can affect people of any age, but it is more common among older adults. Generally, women are more prone to the disease than are men, but among adults younger than 55 men are more likely to develop osteoarthritis.

Signs and Symptoms

One-third of people older than 65 have X-ray evidence of knee osteoarthritis, and 70 percent of people older than 70 have X-ray evidence of osteoarthritis in general. The good news is that just because you show signs of osteoarthritis does not automatically mean you will experience the symptoms of the disease. In fact, only about 50 percent of people who show signs of the disease actually have symptoms. Those symptoms are:

- Pain in one or more joints during or after movement (the joints most often affected are the knees, hips, fingers, lower spine, and neck)

- Stiffness in a joint that is most obvious after a period of inactivity and which lasts no more than 30 minutes

- Tenderness in a joint when you apply light pressure

- Grating or popping sensation you can hear and/or feel when you move the joint

- Development of bone spurs around the affected joint

- Muscle atrophy around the affected joint(s) caused by inactivity

- In knee osteoarthritis, pain exacerbated when moving the knee, pain when standing up, pain when using the stairs, weakening thigh muscles, and a knee that locks or catches

- In hip osteoarthritis pain in the groin, buttocks, or inner thigh and an obvious limp

- In osteoarthritis in the fingers, enlarged joints, painful and swollen finger joints, nodes on the finger joints, and manual dexterity difficulties

- In osteoarthritis of the feet, as pain and tenderness in the big toe (tight shoes and high heels can provoke pain)

- In osteoarthritis of the spine, bone spurs, which occur when disks in the back deteriorate, and pressure on nerves in the spinal cord that causes pain that radiates to the neck, arm, lower back, legs, and/or shoulder

Symptoms of osteoarthritis tend to develop gradually and get worse over time.

DID YOU KNOW?

Knee osteoarthritis is a leading cause of disability in the United States. Approximately 9 million adults were diagnosed with knee osteoarthritis in 2005, and more than half of those affected are older than 65. (American Academy of Orthopaedic Surgeons)

Causes and Risk Factors

What causes osteoarthritis? That's a good question. Even though there is archaeological evidence that arthritis existed millennia ago and despite decades of research, no one has come up with a simple answer to this question. No expert has yet identified why certain joints are affected by osteoarthritis or what causes the cartilage damage that is the trigger for the characteristic wear and tear of the disease.

Although the natural course of aging can contribute to the breakdown in the joints and cause osteoarthritis, not all older people develop the disease. Therefore, experts have identified risk factors for osteoarthritis. These factors fall into two general categories: those over which you have no control and those that you may be able to change or control. The first five risk factors are in the latter category.

- **Age.** Although osteoarthritis can affect people of any age, the risk of developing the disease increases with age. Fifty percent of people older than 65 have osteoarthritis in at least one joint.

- **Ethnicity.** Caucasians have a greater risk of developing osteoarthritis than Asians. African-American women have more knee osteoarthritis and less hand disease than do Caucasian women.

- **Gender.** Among people younger than 45, more men have the disease; among those 55 and older, women are affected more.

- **Family history.** Having a close family member with some form of arthritis increases your risk of getting the disease.

- **Medical history.** Your chances of developing osteoarthritis increase if you have a history of joint injury, joint surgery, joint infection, Paget's disease, a pituitary disorder, gout or pseudogout, congenital weakness or defect in a joint, or hemochromatosis (excess iron disease).

- **Weakness.** Weak thigh muscles increase the risk of developing osteoarthritis of the knee.

- **Overweight/obesity.** Excess weight places increased stress on weight-bearing joints and is a risk for arthritis. Sixty percent of people who are obese are at risk for developing knee osteoarthritis.

- **Joint trauma.** Injury to a joint may increase your chances of developing arthritis in that joint.

- **Infection.** An infection in a joint can result in arthritis in that joint.

- **Repetitive motion.** A job, hobby, or sport that involves repetitive motions may increase the risk of arthritis in the affected joints. For example, baseball pitchers and carpenters may develop motion-related arthritis.

While the risk factors and causes presented here are commonly associated with conventional medicine, other medical models, including Eastern practices such as Ayurvedic medicine and Chinese Traditional Medicine, and naturopathy, bring several other risk factors and causes to the table.

In Ayurvedic medicine, arthritis is attributed to toxins, which are produced by a poor digestive system. These toxins are said to circulate throughout the body and then settle in weak areas, which in many cases include the joints. Ayurvedic treatments for arthritis reflect this approach to the disease and include nutritional and herbal remedies that focus on preventing the accumulation of toxins as well as their elimination.

In Traditional Chinese Medicine (TCM), arthritis is associated with a disruption in the flow of the life force, of qi (chi). To restore this energy flow in the body and thus relieve symptoms of arthritis, TCM therapies employ both acupuncture and herbal remedies, which are discussed in later chapters.

The naturopathic approach to arthritis considers nutritional risk factors and causes. An imbalance of bacteria in the gastrointestinal tract is proposed as one contributing cause; certain foods are also believed to contribute to inflammation. (I discuss the role of diet in chapter 10.) Therefore, naturopathic treatment options take these factors into consideration.

SPOTLIGHT ON RESEARCH

If your knees face outward, you may be at an increased risk for osteoarthritis. This condition is known as varus alignment, and while it resembles bowleggedness, it is not as extreme. According to an August 2010 study released by the U.S. National Institutes of Health and published in the journal *Annals of the Rheumatic Diseases*, people with varus alignment were nearly 1.5 times more likely to develop osteoarthritis than individuals who have a straight-legged stance. The authors of the study note that about 70 percent of the force transmitted to a healthy knee while walking is focused on the inside of the knee. Therefore, if the knee is facing outward, there is greater stress on the inside of the knee, which may increase the risk of osteoarthritis.

Preventing Osteoarthritis

Whether you want to prevent osteoarthritis or you already have the condition but want to help prevent any further damage, here are some suggestions from the Arthritis Foundation. The earlier you start these preventive measures the better, so encourage any young people you know to start *now*!

- **Achieve and maintain ideal body weight.** Any excess weight places unnecessary and harmful stress on your joints.

- **Keep moving!** Exercise to strengthen the muscles around joints and to help prevent deterioration of cartilage in the joints. I discuss different physical exercises and activities in chapter 7.

- **Pay attention to posture.** Proper posture protects the joints from excessive or abnormal pressure. If you have poor posture, you may favor one side of the body or one leg, for example, and place undue stress on the opposite side or the other leg.

- **Spice it up.** Doing the same exercise routine every day not only is boring; it also places repetitive stress on the same joints, which can lead to osteoarthritis. Strength training should be alternated with different aerobic activities.

- **Remember that pain is *not* gain.** Joint pain is a sign that you have overstressed your joint(s). Rest and perhaps some tender loving care (ice, elevation, massage) may be in order as well.

- **Follow safety precautions.** Injuries can lead to osteoarthritis. Wear the proper shoes for your chosen activity, don helmets, wrist pads, and knee protectors when appropriate, and make sure your equipment is always in good operating condition. Do not take unnecessary chances when participating in activities that could lead to injury.

Diagnosis and Treatment

I cover both diagnosis and treatment in much more detail in subsequent chapters, but here is an introduction. Diagnosis of osteoarthritis typically begins with a medical history, a physical examination, and X-rays to determine if there is any joint damage. Bony enlargements of the joints caused by bone spur formation are a sign of osteoarthritis, so your physician will look for nodes (called Heberden's and Bouchard's nodes) on your hands and bunions on your feet.

Although there are no blood tests that diagnose osteoarthritis (see chapter 4), your doctor may do them to exclude other diseases that can cause secondary osteoarthritis (other diseases or conditions that explain the presence of osteoarthritis, such as an injury, congenital abnormality, or another form of arthritis). He or she may also perform arthrocentesis to exclude other causes. This procedure allows the clinician to analyze the fluid in your joint, and it can also provide relief from pain and swelling as well. (A detailed explanation of diagnostic procedures and techniques is provided in chapter 4.)

Treatment of osteoarthritis focuses on relieving and managing symptoms, improving and conserving mobility, and preserving joint function. These goals can be achieved using both over-the-counter and prescription medications (e.g., nonsteroidal anti-inflammatory drugs, painkillers), both oral and topical; injections of corticosteroids or viscosupplementation; lifestyle changes such as weight control, exercise, and diet; herbal and nutritional remedies; physical therapy; and body and energy therapies. Often individuals find that combining two or more of these approaches is most helpful. Surgery is considered a last resort and may include joint replacement. All of these options are discussed in detail in part 2.

BOTTOM LINE

Millions of Americans get up each day to face the challenges of living with osteoarthritis. The first step to living life to the fullest with this disease is to understand what it is, what it can do to your body, and how you can prevent and manage the signs and symptoms to minimize the negative impact they can have on your life.

CHAPTER TWO

Rheumatoid Arthritis, Gout, and More

It may be hard to believe, but there are more than one hundred different types of arthritis and there are even more when you consider all the subtypes. I have already noted the most common type of arthritis, and in this chapter I hope to accomplish two things. One is to explore in some detail the two "other" more common types of arthritis—rheumatoid arthritis and gout—and then round out the trio of arthritis forms most likely to affect you or someone you love. The other is to share some information about a few of the less common forms of arthritis, because it is possible for people who have osteoarthritis, rheumatoid arthritis, or gout to have more than one type of arthritis simultaneously.

RHEUMATOID ARTHRITIS

Approximately 3.1 million adults in the United States have rheumatoid arthritis. Rheumatoid arthritis can affect people of any age, although symptoms typically first appear between 40 and 60 years of age. Nearly three-quarters of those affected are women.

What is Rheumatoid Arthritis?

Rheumatoid arthritis, unlike osteoarthritis, is an autoimmune disorder, which means the immune system incorrectly perceives the body's healthy tissues as foreign and thus attacks them. This case of mistaken identity can impact not only the joints but various organs as well, which is why rheumatoid arthritis is also referred to as a systemic form of arthritis.

Rheumatoid arthritis is a chronic disease that may begin suddenly or gradually; symptoms of pain and swelling of the joints may appear and then suddenly go away for months, or episodes of symptoms may occur every few weeks or months that subside after a few days. This is known as palindromic rheumatism. About 50 percent of people who experience palindromic rheumatism eventually develop chronic rheumatoid arthritis, while the other half continue to have periodic episodes for years. In a small percentage of people, the episodes eventually go away completely.

The joint damage associated with rheumatoid arthritis begins when the lining of the joint (synovium) swells. The inflamed tissue spreads from the synovial membrane and attacks the joint, which causes the synovium to thicken. The inflammatory cells then release enzymes that digest the cartilage and bone, which results in damage to the joint.

Signs and Symptoms

When it comes to signs and symptoms, rheumatoid arthritis can affect any joint, but it typically impacts both sides of the body. That is, if you have rheumatoid arthritis in your right hand, you most likely also have it in your left hand as well. This differs from osteoarthritis.

Symptoms of rheumatoid arthritis include:

• Painful joints

• Swollen joints that may be red

• Joints that are tender when touched

• Joint stiffness in the morning that may last for several hours

• Firm bumps (called rheumatoid nodules) under the skin on your arms

• Fatigue

• Red, puffy hands

• Low-grade fever

• Weight loss and/or loss of appetite

When the disease first begins, it typically affects the smaller joints—those in the hands, wrists, feet, and ankles. As the disease progresses, the knees, shoulders, elbows, hips, jaw, and neck may be affected as well. The severity of symptoms can vary. It is not uncommon to experience periods when the symptoms are worse—called flare-ups or flares—which are then usually followed by periods of remission, when symptoms subside or even disappear for a while, only to return again. Damage can occur to the bone, cartilage, tendons, and ligaments at any time.

Causes/Risk Factors

As I mentioned, rheumatoid arthritis is an autoimmune disease, and experts do not know what causes the process to begin. Some research indicates that genetics have a role, making some individuals more susceptible to environmental factors, such as bacteria or viruses, that trigger the disease process. However, so far no responsible bacteria or viruses have been found.

In addition to rheumatoid arthritis being more prevalent in women and the age of onset being between 40 and 60, other risk factors for the disease include:

- **Family history.** If a family member has rheumatoid arthritis, it increases your risk. Clinicians believe people can inherit a predisposition to rheumatoid arthritis rather than inheriting the disease itself.

- **Genetics.** People who have specific human leukocyte antigen (HLA) genes have a greater chance of developing rheumatoid arthritis than people who do not have the genes. However, everyone who has HLA genes does not develop rheumatoid arthritis, which means having the genes increases susceptibility and other unknown factors are also likely involved.

- **Pregnancy.** Risk for the disease is greater in women who have never been pregnant and in those who have recently given birth.

- **Smoking.** If you smoke cigarettes, you increase your risk; if you quit, you can reduce it.

- **Stress.** Many patients report having had a very
  stressful life event (death of a loved one, lost job,
  divorce) within the six months before the symptoms became apparent

Prevention

So far, scientists have not found a way to prevent rheumatoid arthritis. You can slow progression of the disease,
however, if you begin treatment early in the disease process, which is when much of the damage is done. Treatment options are discussed in part 2.

Diagnosis and Treatment

No single test is available that can definitively diagnose
rheumatoid arthritis. Because the disease can be difficult
to identify, the American College of Rheumatology de-
vised a list of criteria to help physicians with the diagnostic process. We cover the diagnosis of rheumatoid arthritis
in chapter 4. In fact, the good news is that the American
College of Rheumatology, in collaboration with the European League Against Rheumatism, recently (August 2010)
revised the classification criteria for rheumatoid arthritis,
which will now allow the study of treatments for the disease at much earlier stages, even before joint damage occurs, and ultimately leading to better treatments and
improved quality of life for patients.

Early diagnosis is important so treatment can begin
and hopefully stem the advance of the disease. Because
much of the joint damage associated with rheumatoid arthritis occurs during the first two years of the disease, clinicians
generally emphasize early and aggressive treatment. This
approach helps to prevent as much disability as possible. A
wide variety of medications are available to treat this

disease, including nonsteroidal anti-inflammatory drugs, painkillers, disease-modifying antirheumatic drugs, biologic response modifiers, and drug combinations. Alternative body and energy therapies, nutritional therapy, herbal remedies, and other complementary treatments can also be helpful. These are covered in part 2.

GOUT

Gout, also referred to as gouty arthritis, is a condition characterized by an abnormal breakdown (metabolism) of uric acid. When people think of gout, they typically think of the big toe, because that is the joint most commonly affected by this form of arthritis. However, gout can involve other joints besides this single toe. An estimated 3 million people have gout, and some estimates are as high as 5 million, while another 6.1 million have had the disease at some point in their lives. It can occur alone (called primary gout), or it may be associated with another medical condition or use of medication (called secondary gout).

Signs and Symptoms

The first indication that you may have gouty arthritis is the sudden appearance of a hot, red, swollen joint, typically the one at the base of the big toe. Gout that affects this joint is called podagra. The pain can be so intense, merely touching a bedsheet on the affected toe can be excruciating. One sure thing about gout: there is nothing subtle about it!

The first few attacks of gout usually disappear within two weeks, even if you don't treat it. Although it seems to go away, it often returns in the same joint or in another one. With each subsequent attack, the length of the episodes may keep increasing, and they may occur closer and closer together. The number of joints affected each time may also increase.

About 20 percent of people with gout also have urinary tract stones and can develop an interstitial urate nephropathy (rapidly worsening kidney function caused by high levels of uric acid in the urine). They also often develop uric acid crystals, called tophi, that form outside different joints throughout the body, such as the elbow, Achilles tendon, and earlobe. Although tophi usually are not painful, they can be a clue for the diagnosis of gout if your doctor removes them with a needle for examination under a microscope.

Causes/Risk Factors

Gout is caused by the accumulation of excess uric acid in the body. Uric acid is a by-product of the metabolism of a substance called purine, which is found in food and in all human tissues. If the body produces too much uric acid (which is the case in 10 percent of people who have gout) or the kidneys cannot eliminate it (90 percent of cases), the buildup of uric acid results in the development of crystals that are deposited in the joints. These crystals trigger inflammation. Repeated "attacks" of gouty arthritis can result in chronic inflammation, damage the affected joint(s), and lead to osteoarthritis. The good news is that although gout is a progressive disease, there are several effective medications and other treatment options to deal with this form of arthritis.

There are many risk factors for gouty arthritis:

- **Sex.** Males are about nine times more likely to get gout than women. Gouty arthritis is also considered to be the most common cause of inflammatory arthritis in men older than 40. Women are more likely to develop gout after menopause.

• **Family history.** About 20 percent of people with gout have a family history of the disease.

• **Certain groups.** American blacks (but not African blacks) are more likely to develop gout than whites, and the British are five times more likely to develop gout. The reason for this is unknown.

• **Overweight/obesity.** Excess weight means there is an abundance of tissue that can break down, which results in excess production of uric acid.

• **Alcohol use.** Drinking alcohol not only increases uric acid production; it also hinders the elimination of uric acid from the body. Beer is the main culprit among alcoholic beverages.

• **Purines.** Eating foods rich in purines is a risk factor for gout. Examples of such foods include dried beans, organ meats, pork, beef, poultry, fish, and alcohol.

• **Concomitant conditions.** People who have the following disorders or ailments are at greater risk of developing gout: psoriasis, diabetes, high blood pressure, sarcoidosis, Down syndrome, hypothyroidism, diabetic ketoacidosis, preeclampsia, kidney disorders (e.g., renal insufficiency, polycystic kidney disease).

- **Lead exposure.** Being exposed to lead either at work or through lead-based paint or other environmental means can increase your risk.

- **Organ transplant.** Transplant recipients are at greater risk for gout.

- **Certain medications.** If you take any of the following medications, it increases your risk of developing gout: diuretics, salicylates, niacin, cyclosporine, levodopa, nicotinic acid, allopurinol, or probenecid.

- **Enzyme defect.** Some conditions, such as glucose-6-phosphatase deficiency and fructose-1-phosphate deficiency, make it difficult for the body to break down purines.

- **Kidney disease.** A diseased kidney is less able to eliminate uric acid, and thus increases the risk of developing gout.

- **Sudden elevation of uric acid levels.** This can be caused by trauma, starvation, dehydration, use of intravenous contrast dyes, or chemotherapy.

Prevention

After looking at the list of risk factors for gout, you may be saying to yourself, *Wow, what can I do to help prevent it?* Although the list of preventive measures may not be as long as the one of risk factors, it is well worth considering.

- Follow a low-cholesterol, low-fat diet. This approach lowers your risk of both gout and heart disease. (See chapter 10.)

- Avoid foods that are high in purines, as I mentioned in the risk factor list.

- If you are on a weight-loss regimen, lose weight slowly. Losing weight rapidly can sometimes stimulate an attack of gout.

- Avoid foods that contain fructose and corn syrup.

- Stay hydrated.

- Limit your intake of alcohol, especially beer.

- If you are taking thiazide diuretics, levodopa, cyclosporine, nicotinic acid, or aspirin, talk to your doctor about alternatives.

Diagnosis and Treatment

Along with the typical medical history, physical examination, and discussion of your symptoms, your doctor may also take a fluid sample from the affected joint and/ or a blood sample. More details about the diagnosis of gout are found in chapter 4.

Treatment of gouty arthritis may consist of one or more medications, along with suggested changes to your diet. A variety of treatment options are explored in part 2 of this book, including a gout diet in chapter 10.

CATEGORIES OF ARTHRITIS

Inflammatory types of arthritis are those that involve the immune system and the presence of inflammatory white blood cells in the fluid around the affected joint. Many forms of inflammatory arthritis are autoimmune disorders, which means the body recognizes its own tissues as invaders and attacks them, resulting in inflammation. Inflammatory arthritis can also be caused by bacteria or deposits of crystalline structures in the joints. Forms of inflammatory arthritis include rheumatoid arthritis, lupus, gout, ankylosing spondylitis, and many others.

Noninflammatory arthritis is a form in which the symptoms are provoked by movement and activities and then improve and calm down after rest. Osteoarthritis, the most common type of arthritis, falls into this category, along with arthritis of thyroid disease, neuropathic arthropathy, and others.

Infectious arthritis (also known as septic arthritis) is an infection in a joint that is most often caused by bacteria or viruses but can also be the result of a fungus or parasite. A large single joint such as the knee or hip is usually targeted, but multiple joints can be infected as well. Infectious arthritis is considered a medical emergency because it can cause serious damage to the bone and cartilage. Infectious arthritis, which includes tuberculosis arthritis, viral arthritis, and reactive arthritis, affects about twenty thousand people per year. People with a history of arthritis are more likely to develop infectious arthritis.

OTHER TYPES OF ARTHRITIS

The 10 types of arthritis explained here were chosen based on their prevalence and, in some cases, because they can occur along with any of the three main forms of arthritis I discuss throughout the book. For more information about any of these and other types of arthritis, see "Resources" in the back of this book.

Ankylosing Spondylitis

Ankylosing (means "fusion") spondylitis (inflammation of a spinal joint) is a chronic inflammatory disease that often attacks the spine, specifically the sacroiliac joints at the base, and can cause the vertebrae to fuse together. It can also impact the hips, knees, and shoulders, as well as the ligaments and tendons around the bones and joints. Approximately 350,000 people in the United States have ankylosing spondylitis. It is three times more prevalent in men than women, and the disease usually first appears between ages 15 and 40.

The first indication of ankylosing spondylitis is lower back pain that comes and goes. As the disease progresses, pain and stiffness may spread beyond the sacroiliac joints to affect more of the spine. Other signs and symptoms may include an inability to fully expand the chest because the joints between the ribs are affected, heel and/or hip pain, fatigue, and eye inflammation.

The course of the disease is unpredictable: symptoms can appear and then disappear at any time. Most people can function well unless their hips are severely affected. As the disease progresses, the body forms new bone, which causes the vertebrae to grow together, forming vertical bony outgrowths that become stiff and inflexible. This is the type of fusion that can stiffen the rib cage and restrict lung capacity.

Most people who have ankylosing spondylitis have the HLA-B27 gene. Having the gene makes people more susceptible to the disease but does not guarantee they will get it. Except for the presence of the HLA-B27 gene, there are no known specific causes of ankylosing spondylitis.

Bursitis and Tendinitis

Bursitis is inflammation or irritation of the bursae, fluid-filled sacs that can be found between tissues such as muscle, tendons, skin, and bone. These sacs help decrease friction, rubbing, and other irritation, but when they become inflamed, usually by repetitive activity or overuse (e.g., engaging in golf, gardening, tennis, raking, carpentry, pitching) or a sudden injury, the result is pain. Loss of motion in the shoulder, called frozen shoulder, can also be a sign of bursitis.

Bursitis is more common in adults older than 40 and most often affects the elbow, shoulder, hip, knee, or Achilles tendon. Stress or inflammation from rheumatoid arthritis or gout can also increase a person's risk of developing bursitis. Treatment can include anti-inflammatory medications, steroids, physical therapy, icing the area, and rest.

Tendinitis is inflammation or irritation of a tendon, which also is often caused by repetitive motion and the same types of activities associated with bursitis. Stress from other conditions, including rheumatoid arthritis and gout, is a risk factor for tendinitis. Occasionally an infection can cause tendinitis.

Tendinitis most often occurs in the elbow, base of the thumb, shoulder, hip, knee, and Achilles tendon. Adults older than 40 are most often affected, and as with bursitis, pain and frozen shoulder are common symptoms. Treatment for tendinitis is much the same as for bursitis.

Carpal Tunnel Syndrome

Many people think of carpal tunnel syndrome as a condition that most affects individuals who spend hours working on a computer keyboard or as cashiers. But this form of arthritis is common among carpenters, mechanics, painters, artists, golfers, knitters, car drivers, dishwashers, tennis players, and others. Conditions that are associated with carpal tunnel syndrome and contribute to its development include rheumatoid arthritis, tendinitis, obesity, aging, diabetes, and cysts.

The carpal tunnel is a narrow passageway located on the palm side of your wrist that is bound by ligaments and bones. Its job is to protect a main nerve to your hand and nine tendons that allow you to bend your fingers. When pressure is placed on the nerve—which can come from repetitive use that leads to swelling, conditions such as rheumatoid arthritis or fluid retention due to pregnancy, or because you have an abnormally narrow carpal tunnel—it results in pain, numbness, tingling, and hand weakness that can eventually extend to the forearm. If the condition is not treated, it can lead to nerve and muscle damage. Treatment can include splinting the wrist, icing and resting the wrist, and use of nonsteroidal anti-inflammatory drugs or corticosteroids. Surgery usually results in significant improvement in about 70 percent of patients, but

some people experience some residual numbness, stiffness, weakness, or pain.

Fibromyalgia

Do you hurt all over, feel tired most of the time, and no doctor seems to know what's wrong with you? You may have
fibromyalgia, a chronic condition characterized by widespread pain in the muscles, tendons, and ligaments, along
with fatigue and many places called tender points where
slight pressure causes pain. Between 10 and 15 percent of
people who have osteoarthritis also have fibromyalgia, and
people who have rheumatoid arthritis or lupus are also more
likely to develop fibromyalgia. Overall about 2 percent of
people in the United States have fibromyalgia and women
are much more likely to have the disorder than are men.

Along with widespread pain that lasts three months or
longer, the American College of Rheumatology has determined that a diagnosis of fibromyalgia also requires that
pain be present in 11 of 18 tender points. Other symptoms
associated with the syndrome include headache, sleep
disturbances, irritable bowel or bladder, jaw pain, restless
legs syndrome, sensitivity to cold and heat, depression,
hearing and vision problems, and cognitive difficulties.

No cause of fibromyalgia has been identified, although
symptoms sometimes begin after emotional or physical
trauma. Researchers believe the chronic pain may be
caused by repeated nerve stimulation in the brain, which
causes an abnormal increase in the level of certain brain
chemicals (neurotransmitters) that signal pain.

Lupus

Lupus is a chronic autoimmune disease that can damage
any part of the body, inside and out—skin, bones, joints,

nervous system, and other organs. The Lupus Foundation of America estimates that 1.5 million Americans have a form of lupus. Although it can affect males and females of all ages, 90 percent of cases occur in women. Lupus commonly develops between the ages of 18 and 45.

Lupus appears in a number of different forms. Systemic lupus erythematosus (SLE) accounts for about 70 percent of cases of lupus; the other main types are cutaneous lupus erythematosus (affects only the skin) and drug-induced lupus, which is caused by the use of certain prescription drugs.

Because SLE can affect the entire body, the list of signs and symptoms can be quite extensive. Some of the more common ones are arthritis in multiple joints, rash, fatigue, sores in the mouth and nose, seizures, chest pain or heartburn, sensitivity to sunlight, hair loss, and weight loss. SLE is also associated with serious complications, including inflammation of the kidneys (lupus nephritis), increased blood pressure in the lungs (pulmonary hypertension), inflammation of the nervous system and brain, inflammation in the brain's blood vessels, and coronary artery disease.

No one has identified the cause of lupus, although one popular theory is that people are born with the genes that make them susceptible and then something triggers the disease and its symptoms. Because the disease is so prevalent in women, hormones are believed to have a role as well.

Lyme Disease

The bite of a common deer tick is the trigger for Lyme disease, an arthritis-related condition that is caused by the bacterium *Borrelia burgdorferi,* which is carried by the tick. Lyme disease is characterized by flu-like symptoms, including joint pain, fatigue, muscle aches, chills, fever, swollen lymph nodes, and headache. In 70 to 80 percent of people, a rash that resembles a bull's-eye appears around the tick bite.

Several weeks after being bitten by an infected tick, 60 percent of people develop recurrent attacks of swollen and painful joints if they have not been treated with antibiotics. About 10 to 20 percent of untreated patients develop lasting arthritis, and osteoarthritis frequently occurs in people who have lupus.

Treatment with appropriate antibiotics early during the course of the disease is usually effective in eliminating the disease. In more serious cases, intravenous antibiotics may be necessary. Most people respond well to antibiotics and recovery fully. Some patients, however, have persistent symptoms. If not treated, Lyme disease can cause permanent damage to the joints, nervous system, and heart. Lyme disease can strike more than once in the same person if he or she is bitten by another infected tick.

Polymyalgia Rheumatica

Polymyalgia rheumatica, which means "many muscle pains" and "changing," is an inflammatory condition that causes pain or aching in the large muscle groups, especially around the hips and shoulders. It typically affects people older than 50 and is more common in women than men. Because many other conditions have signs and symptoms similar to those of polymyalgia rheumatica, it can be a challenge to diagnose. The good news, however, is that it is very treatable.

In addition to muscle pain, symptoms of polymyalgia rheumatica include weakness, fatigue, generally feeling ill, weight loss, and stiffness around the hips and shoulders, especially in the morning. About 15 percent of people with polymylagia rheumatica also have temporal arteritis, which is inflammation of the arteries, especially those that provide blood to the head and temples. Headache is the most common symptom.

Blood tests are typically used to help diagnose polymyalgia rheumatica and to rule out other possible causes of the symptoms, such as rheumatoid arthritis or hypothyroidism. Steroids are a common treatment for this disease, although long-term use of these drugs can result in heart and lung problems, diabetes, and bone loss.

Psoriatic Arthritis

Like rheumatoid arthritis, psoriatic arthritis is an inflammatory form of arthritis, and in this case it combines chronic joint pain and the skin disease psoriasis. About 15 percent of people who have the skin disease psoriasis go on to develop psoriatic arthritis. About 1 million Americans have psoriatic arthritis, and it affects men and women equally.

In 85 percent of people who develop psoriatic arthritis, symptoms of psoriasis appear first. There are five types of psoriatic arthritis, characterized by symptoms, but the most common type is asymmetric psoriatic arthritis. This form of psoriatic arthritis can affect any joint in the body, and swollen sausage-like fingers and toes are common. Psoriatic arthritis is usually treated with the same medications used to treat rheumatoid arthritis.

Scleroderma

Scleroderma is an autoimmune, arthritis-related condition that is actually a symptom of a group of diseases that are complicated by the abnormal growth of connective tissue that supports the skin and other organs. There are two major types of scleroderma: localized scleroderma, which mainly affects the skin and is characterized by hard or thickened skin; and systemic scleroderma, which can affect the internal organs. Approximately seventy-five to one hundred thousand people in the United States have scleroderma. It most often affects women between the ages of 30 and 50, but it can develop in children and men as well.

The first sign of scleroderma is often Raynaud's phenomenon, in which the small blood vessels narrow in the fingers, toes, ear, and nose. Attacks of Raynaud's phenomenon can occur several times daily and are often triggered by exposure to cold. First pitted scars appear on the hands, and then the skin on the hands, feet, and face thickens and hardens. Patches of thick, hardened skin may develop on other areas of the body as well. The skin can continue to worsen for several years, and then the disease may go into remission and the skin may improve. Eventually, however, the disease progresses and the skin loses its ability to stretch.

Patients also experience changes in bones, muscles, and joints. Mild arthritis typically affects both sides of the body, and there can be bone destruction similar to that seen in rheumatoid arthritis. Individuals can have difficulty bending their fingers if the disease affects the tendons and joints. Hypertension, heartburn, and other symptoms may also occur.

Some people with scleroderma also experience gastrointestinal disorders, lung scarring (pulmonary fibrosis), scarring of the heart (fibrosis), and kidney problems. While there is no treatment that can prevent the skin thickening that is characteristic of the disease, medications are usually prescribed for the arthritis, hypertension, and other consequences of scleroderma.

Sjogren's Syndrome

Sjogren's syndrome is an inflammatory autoimmune disease that primarily attacks the tear and saliva glands, which results in dry eyes and dry mouth. Other body parts can also be affected. The syndrome can be either primary or secondary. Primary Sjogren's occurs without the presence of other connective tissue or autoimmune diseases, while secondary Sjogren's occurs with rheumatic diseases such as rheumatoid arthritis, lupus, and scleroderma. About 50 percent of people with Sjogren's syndrome have secondary Sjogren's. Overall, between 2 and 4 million Americans are affected by Sjogren's syndrome and 90 percent of them are women.

Along with the two most common symptoms of dry eyes and dry mouth, Sjogren's syndrome is also characterized by dry nose, throat, and lungs, vaginal dryness, fatigue, dental problems, and swollen salivary glands. In more severe cases, confusion, muscle weakness, memory problems, and feelings of numbness and tingling can develop. The cause of Sjogren's syndrome is not known, although genetics, hormones, and infections are all suspect. Symptoms are usually treated with medications typically used for other forms of arthritis, including nonsteroidal anti-inflammatory drugs and disease-modifying antirheumatic drugs in more severe cases.

THE COMPLETE REALM OF ARTHRITIS

Arthritis and arthritis-related conditions is a broad category, and from this small sampling I hope you can better understand and appreciate the many facets of arthritis and why it can be challenging for health-care professionals to diagnose these conditions. I have also tried to offer a glimpse into the possibility of you or a loved one having more than one type of arthritis. For a complete list of the different types of arthritis and arthritis-related conditions, see "100-plus Types of Arthritis" at the back of this book.

Now that I have mentioned health-care professionals, it is time to investigate how to go about finding providers who can best help you with a diagnosis and treatment of the signs and symptoms of arthritis, and help you live the best life you can with arthritis.

CHAPTER THREE

Finding Health-Care Professionals

When you have a chronic condition such as arthritis, you need to find a doctor who will work with you in the long haul, someone you trust and respect, and with whom you can establish a good doctor-patient relationship. Such a relationship will allow you to feel comfortable talking about issues that have a significant impact on your life with arthritis, including decisions about losing weight, stopping smoking, changing your diet, or getting a referral for a therapist so you can tackle symptoms of depression. This type of doctor-patient relationship should be based on mutual respect and understanding. Finding such a doctor does not always happen with your first choice.

Similarly, if you decide at some point you want to consult a nutritionist, naturopath, physical therapist, or other health-care professional, you need to know how to find the one who will work best for you. This chapter helps you find the health-care providers who will help you manage arthritis, explore new possible treatment options with you, and ultimately help you improve and maintain your health while living with arthritis. I realize that given health insurance limitations and perhaps the lack of health insurance, your options may be reduced, yet it is still possible to choose the most compatible health-care provider from those available to you.

WHERE TO BEGIN

If you are looking for a doctor to diagnose, treat, and manage your arthritis, put away your phone book and set aside your health plan's list of physicians. According to a recent Consumer Reports survey, people who found their doctor by getting a recommendation from someone they trusted, such as a friend, family member, or another doctor, were the most pleased with their choice. If you can get several recommendations, hopefully at least one of them will be on your insurance carrier's list, if you are indeed limited to a list of physicians.

Generalist or Specialist?

The general recommendation is to have a primary care doctor who takes care of your routine health needs, such as examinations and treatment of common problems such as flu or strep throat. He or she can be a family practice physician or a general internist and should coordinate any care you receive from specialists for arthritis or other complicated conditions.

You may also get both your primary care and your specialty care from a specialized physician. For example, you may want your rheumatologist (the specialist many people with arthritis turn to for their care). You need to make sure, however, that he or she will do the more generalized care typically performed by a primary care physician.

Rheumatologist

Since I brought up a rheumatologist, let's begin with this specialty. Rheumatologists are physicians who specialize in rheumatic diseases, which include the three I am focusing on in this book: osteoarthritis, rheumatoid arthritis, and gout, among other types of arthritis. Rheumatology is a subspecialty of internal medicine, which means the physician must have completed three years in internal or pediatric medicine beyond the four years at medical school, plus two to three years of specialized education and training in rheumatic diseases and treatment. At that point, the rheumatologist candidates must pass exams to become certified by the American Board of Internal Medicine.

If at all possible, I suggest you find a rheumatologist to help you with your arthritis. He or she can conduct your examinations, interpret your test results, prescribe treatment options, suggest further investigations from other specialists, and refer you for surgery if necessary.

If you need help finding a rheumatologist in your area, you can ask your primary care physician for a referral, ask friends and family members, or contact the American College of Rheumatology (www.rheumatology.org) and their Web site, which provides information on how to locate rheumatologists in all areas of the United States.

Orthopedic Surgeon

I hope you will never need this specialist, but if you do, there are more than twenty-five thousand orthopedic surgeons practicing in the United States from whom to choose, according to the American Academy of Orthopaedic Surgeons (AAOS). If you need joint surgery, an orthopedic surgeon is the specialist you will want to turn to. These doctors perform joint replacement surgery and other joint-related operations on patients who have osteo-arthritis, rheumatoid arthritis, or gout that has not responded to other therapeutic methods.

Adult knee surgery is the most popular subspecialty within the field of orthopedics. Thirty-four percent of orthopedic surgeons practice in this subspecialty area, while another 34 percent specialize in arthroscopy and 33 percent list sports medicine as their specialty. (Note: some surgeons specialize in more than one area.) The *Orthopaedic Practice in the U.S. 2008* report notes that orthopedic surgeons perform an average of 32 orthopedic procedures per month. Therefore when looking for a surgeon, keep this number in mind. You will want a surgeon who regularly performs the type of surgery you are planning.

At the 2009 AAOS Annual Meeting, two studies were presented, each of which warned that the number of patients who would be seeking hip or knee replacement surgery was expected to quickly outpace the number of orthopedic surgeons available to perform the procedures. In fact, the research indicated that by 2016 there would not be enough physicians to complete 46 percent of the needed hip replacements and 72 percent of the needed knee replacements.

If you ever need a knee or hip replacement, or another type of orthopedic surgery for arthritis, there are many professionals from whom to choose. For details about the surgical procedures these professionals can perform for patients who have arthritis, see chapter 9.

Physical Therapist

Physical therapists diagnose and treat people of all ages who have health-related conditions or medical problems that limit their abilities to move and perform regular daily functional activities. Your doctor may refer you to a physical therapist or a physical therapy clinic where you will likely find several professionals from whom to choose. However, most states allow you to go directly to a physical therapist without a doctor's referral. In either case, you need to check with your insurance provider, because some require that you visit a primary care physician first or may limit your choice to only preferred providers. Physical therapists practice in hospitals, private practices, outpatient clinics, rehabilitation facilities, skilled nursing facilities, homes, schools, and athletic facilities.

When choosing a physical therapist, only consider one who is licensed. Each state has its own licensing requirements for physical therapists. If you are receiving physical therapy from a physical therapist assistant, make sure he or she is supervised by a licensed physical therapist.

Physical therapists must have a graduate degree from an accredited physical therapy program before they take the national licensure examination. The minimum educational requirement for physical therapists is a master's degree, although some go on to get the doctor of physical therapy (DPT) degree.

CHECK UP ON YOUR DOCTOR

Your doctor does a checkup on you, but you can do the same on him or her. Several services—some free, some requiring a fee—provide information on licensing, disciplinary actions, board certification, educational history, and/or hospital admitting privileges for physicians. Here are six services you can access. The first three provide free information.

- **Administrators in Medicine (www.docboard.org/docfinder.html).** This service offers information on licensing and disciplinary actions taken against physicians (and osteopaths) in 21 states. There are links to state medical boards of the remaining states.

- **American Board of Medical Specialties** (www. abms.org). Is your doctor certified in his or her specialty? This site will help you discover the answer. Board certification means the individual has completed an approved residency program and passed a specialized written exam in at least 1 of 24 specialty areas, such as internal medicine.

- **American Medical Association DoctorFinder (webapps.ama-assn.org/doctorfinder).** This service provides comprehensive information on doctors, including their educational background, hospital admitting privileges, and board certification for about 40 percent of the physicians who belong to the AMA.

- **Consumers' CHECKBOOK Guide to Top Doctors (www.checkbook.org).** This service charges a fee, for which you get access to a searchable database of the top-ranked doctors in 30 fields based on a survey of more than 260,000 physicians.

- **HealthGrades** **(www.healthgrades.com).** This service provides reports on doctors for a fee, including education and training, board certification, professional misconduct or disciplinary actions, and satisfaction scores from patients.

- **Your state board of medicine.** You can contact your state board to learn if a doctor has been fined or had his/her license suspended or revoked. (Or ask someone at your county courthouse for information on lost malpractice suits.)

YOUR ROLE IN THE DOCTOR-PATIENT RELATIONSHIP

For the best quality care and satisfaction, you should not be a passive partner in the doctor-patient relationship. If you take an active part in your diagnosis and treatment, you are more likely to be satisfied with the results. Therefore, your role in the doctor-patient relationship is to keep records of your symptoms and related information, ask questions of your health-care providers, and be alert to new studies and research findings so you can ask your providers if new information can benefit you.

Let's start with records. You can best help your doctor help you by keeping records of changes in your symptoms as well as any reactions to foods, medications, supplements, or other factors. One way to achieve this is by keeping a symptoms diary.

Symptoms Diary

A symptoms diary can be as elaborate or as simple as you want it to be, just as long as it helps you keep track of information that may prove useful for your doctor. Some people keep a symptoms diary much like they would a regular diary, writing in narrative style. Others jot down notes on different key areas, such as a description of their symptoms and rating them from 0 to 10, when the symptom occurred, if medications were taken, response to the medication, and possible triggers (e.g., foods, weather). You can even formalize your notes by preparing a chart with these categories, making enough copies for several weeks or months, and filling one in each day. You will then have an accurate record of your symptoms to discuss with your health-care provider.

Questions, Questions, Questions!

When you are looking for a physician, there are questions you need to ask yourself as well as those you should ask the doctor. Here are some you should consider in both categories. First, ask yourself:

- Do I prefer to work with a male or female doctor? It is important to feel comfortable with the doctor you choose and to feel like you can talk about your health concerns without feeling embarrassed.

- Do I want my doctor to be younger, older, or about my age?

- Do I have a preference for a doctor based on language and/or culture?

- Do I have a preference as to where the doctor received his/her education?

Now, here are some questions you can ask the doctor and the doctor's staff and/or discover on your own:

- Is the doctor board certified?

- Where does the doctor have hospital privileges?

- What is the average wait during appointments?

- Is the doctor's office in a convenient location, and

does the doctor have office hours that fit your lifestyle or work schedule?

• Does the doctor accept your insurance?

• If you are looking for an orthopedic surgeon, does the doctor have FACS (Fellow of the American College of Surgeons) after his/her name?

• Is the doctor part of a group practice? If your doctor was not available, would you be asked to see his/her colleague? Is this something with which you are comfortable?

• How does the doctor feel about alternative/complementary treatments, including the use of nutritional supplements and herbs?

• Is the office staff helpful and friendly?

Have you chosen a candidate? Now is the time to make an appointment for your initial consultation and your physical exam. Before you walk into the office, you should prepare a list of questions to help you make your final decision. You may want to bring along a family member, partner, or friend for moral support. Another person's perspective on the doctor and the interchange between you and the doctor can be invaluable when you are making your final decision. After your initial visit, you can think about:

• Did the doctor answer your questions to your satisfaction?

• Did the doctor seem to really care about you and your concerns?

• Did you feel comfortable during the consultation and examination?

BOTTOM LINE

I realize that your insurance plan may not provide you with a large pool of doctors from whom to choose or you may not have insurance and have limited options. However, these challenges do not mean you cannot be proactive—ask questions, learn as much as you can about the doctors who are available, and keep good records so you can provide the information to the doctor you do choose.

CHAPTER FOUR

Getting a Diagnosis

Before you can begin the right treatment for your symptoms, you need an accurate diagnosis. Some people are under the impression that getting a diagnosis of arthritis is an easy task: one quick visit to your doctor and you can walk out with a prescription for medications to take care of your symptoms. However, because there are so many different types of arthritis and so many of the signs and symptoms are the same as those of other conditions, the road to an accurate diagnosis can be a challenging one. Indeed, some people who have been rather offhandedly diagnosed with arthritis—or diagnosed themselves— eventually discover that either they have a different type of arthritis than they believed or they do not have arthritis at all but another condition that has mimicked many of the symptoms.

But you can help your doctor by being prepared for your appointments. In this chapter I help you prepare for the diagnostic process by explaining what questions you need to ask, which questions will be asked of you, what information you can gather before you go to your appointment (including a symptoms diary), and what to expect from your doctor during the diagnostic process.

Diagnosing arthritis always begins with the standard

review of your personal and family medical history, a review of your current symptoms and health status, and then a physical examination. In this chapter I discuss these steps as well as the different tests your doctor may order (e.g., blood and urine tests, imaging) and what the results can mean. When you're through with this chapter, you will know what to expect from your doctor and hopefully feel secure about the process.

DIAGNOSING OSTEOARTHRITIS

Your doctor has already gathered your personal and family medical history, and so now it's time for the next step. During the physical examination part of your visit, your doctor will

- Press on your joints. In people who have osteoarthritis, the affected joint will generally be tender when pressure is applied right along the joint line.

- Move your joints in different directions to determine your range of motion and whether movement causes pain.

- Listen to see if he or she hears any clicking or grating noise when your joints are moved. Such sounds are common in people who have osteoarthritis. Often people who have arthritis in their spine, for example, will say they can hear (and feel) a crackling sound when they bend or twist a certain way.

- Examine your joints to determine if they are swollen, deformed, or enlarged. The bones around the affected joints may feel larger than normal, and the joint's range of motion is often reduced. Normal movement of the joint is often painful.

Your doctor may also calculate your body mass index (BMI), which is a measurement of your body fat based on your height and weight. Being overweight or obese can have a significant impact on joint pain, and so your doctor may encourage you to lose weight.

Questions Your Doctor May Ask

Before or during your physical examination, your doctor may ask the following questions:

- Do you experience pain at night?

- Which joints are painful and how long have they been bothering you?

- When does the pain start? Is the pain associated with certain physical activities? Does it improve after you rest?

- Are your joints stiff when you wake up in the morning? If yes, how long does the stiffness last?

- Do your joints ever lock up or give out (e.g., do your knees buckle)?

- Do you have a family history of osteoarthritis?

- Are you currently taking any medications or supplements to treat your symptoms?

A telltale sign of osteoarthritis is often identifiable on X-rays. Specifically, your doctor will likely see cartilage loss suggested by certain characteristics, such as a narrowed space between the bones in a joint, an abnormal increase in bone density, and the presence of bony projections (e.g., bone spurs or osteophytes), cysts, or erosion.

While X-rays are a valuable diagnostic tool for osteoarthritis, it is important to note that you can still have the disease even if your X-rays do not show any abnormalities. Similarly, some people experience minimal or mild symptoms of osteoarthritis even though their X-rays clearly show bone and joint problems. If your doctor suspects there may be other reasons for your pain, he or she may also order an MRI of an arthritic joint (see "Magnetic Resonance Imaging").

DID YOU KNOW?

Bone spurs, or osteophytes, are common in people who have arthritis. These bony projections form along joints and can greatly limit joint motion while also causing pain. Bone spurs form when the body makes an attempt to increase the surface area of the joint to better distribute weight across a joint, especially a knee or hip, that has been damaged by arthritis. Unfortunately, this attempt to remedy a problem creates another one—a bone spur.

DIAGNOSING RHEUMATOID ARTHRITIS

As of August 2010, rheumatologists had at their disposal the official diagnostic criteria for rheumatoid arthritis as determined by the American College of Rheumatology, which established the guidelines in 1987. According to these criteria, an official diagnosis of rheumatoid arthritis is given when four or more of these seven factors are present. The first four factors must have been present for at least six weeks.

1. Morning stiffness in and around the joints for at least one hour
2. Swelling or accumulation of fluid around three or more joints simultaneously
3. At least one swollen area in the hand, finger joints, or wrist
4. Arthritis that involves the same joint on both sides of the body
5. Presence of rheumatoid nodules, which are usually found in pressure points, most often the elbows
6. Abnormal amounts of rheumatoid factor in the blood
7. X-ray evidence in the hands and wrists of rheumatoid arthritis that includes destruction of bone around the involved joints

Along with a medical history and physical examination, clinicians order blood tests to look for factors that can help with diagnosis, including rheumatoid factor, erythrocyte sedimentation rate, C-reactive protein, and anti-CCP tests. X-rays and magnetic resonance imaging may be used to identify joint damage (see details on these tests later in this chapter).

The (Near) Future of Diagnosing Rheumatoid Arthritis

In August 2010, the American College of Rheumatology, along with the European League Against Rheumatism, established a new set of classification criteria that will serve as the basis for the development of new diagnostic criteria for rheumatoid arthritis that can be used by rheumatologists in their practices. As of this writing, however, those new diagnostic criteria had not been determined.

By way of a "sneak" preview, the investigators who worked on the new classification criteria revealed that for a patient to be classified as having "definite RA," he or she must get a score of 6 or higher, out of a possible 10. Alan Silman, M.D., who initiated the project, explained that the scoring system takes into account the results of lab tests for inflammation and autoimmunity, the number, location, and size of involved joints, and how long patients have had their symptoms. Patients should also have confirmed synovitis—inflammation of the synovial membranes that line the joint—in at least one joint, and the cause of the synovitis should not be explained by another diagnosis, such as gout.

Stanley B. Cohen, M.D., president of the American College of Rheumatology, noted that the new classification criteria would "open the door to more meaningful studies of RA and will eventually lead to changes in the diagnosis and treatment of the disease. This is an important step for RA researchers, practicing rheumatologists and patients."

The Challenge of Diagnosing Rheumatoid Arthritis

Rheumatoid arthritis can be finicky, as symptoms can come and go. To make an accurate diagnosis, your doctor may need to examine you when the disease is in its active stage. One reason is that symptoms of rheumatoid arthritis can appear similar to other common causes of joint pain, so trying to make a diagnosis when the disease is dormant may lead to a wrong diagnosis. Some of the other common causes include osteoarthritis, fibromyalgia, joint inflammation caused by an infection, and gout.

Another reason is that many patients find it difficult to describe their symptoms to their doctor in a way that is helpful to the physician. However, if you keep a symptoms diary, this hurdle can be overcome! Unfortunately, many people do not keep accurate records, and for this reason and others the average time between when symptoms begin and an individual gets an official diagnosis of rheumatoid arthritis is nearly nine months.

The main reason it is so important to accurately diagnose rheumatoid arthritis as early as possible is that joint damage can occur in the beginning stages of the disease. Delaying a diagnosis can result in serious, permanent damage. Making a misdiagnosis, however, is also not safe, because the medications typically used to treat the disease are powerful and can have serious side effects. Therefore, it is important that you keep a symptoms diary or something similar, because it can make a big difference in your diagnosis and treatment. If you suspect you have rheumatoid arthritis and you have not seen a doctor, make an appointment as soon as possible.

DIAGNOSING GOUT

Although most people think of gout as being a big pain in the big toe, it takes a bit more investigation to make a firm diagnosis. The most definitive test to diagnose gout is joint aspiration, as it also rules out other causes of pain and inflammation, such as an infection in the joint. To perform aspiration, your doctor will insert a needle into the affected joint and withdraw a fluid sample for testing. He or she will look for gout crystals or signs of a bacterial infection in the fluid. In some cases, your doctor may find other crystals in the fluid, such as calcium pyrophosphate, which is caused by a different condition called pseudogout ("like gout").

In some cases, doctors may use a blood sample to evaluate your cell counts, kidney function, and uric acid levels. However, a uric acid level is not a reliable resource to make a diagnosis of gout, because levels can be normal in approximately 10 percent of people during an acute attack of gouty arthritis. In addition, uric acid levels are elevated in about 5 to 8 percent of the general population, so a high uric level does not automatically mean that gout is the cause of a person's inflamed joint. To make diagnosis even more challenging, the uric acid level is typically lowered during a flare-up of inflammatory gouty arthritis. Therefore the best time to measure uric acid is after a flare-up has subsided and when acute inflammation has disappeared.

In some cases, a doctor may order X-rays if he or she needs to assess underlying joint damage, especially if you have had multiple episodes of gouty arthritis.

PSEUDOGOUT

About 25 percent of the adult population has a condition called pseudogout, also known as chondrocalcinosis. In this disease, a specific type of calcium crystals known as calcium pyrophosphate dehydrate (CPPD) accumulate in the joints. If you already have osteoarthritis, pseudogout can make those symptoms worse. A doctor can usually tell the difference between osteoarthritis and pseudogout because the latter usually damages joints that are not normally affected by osteoarthritis, such as wrists, elbows, and shoulders.

TESTS AND PROCEDURES

X-rays

X-rays can reveal localized bone loss, which means bone erosion, a characteristic of rheumatoid arthritis. Clinicians can also use X-rays to identify osteoarthritis, which can be characterized by the presence of bone spurs (also known as osteophytes) and loss of joint space. Doctors also use X-rays to help them decide whether a patient is a good candidate for joint replacement surgery.

Magnetic Resonance Imaging

Magnetic resonance imaging can be helpful in diagnosing arthritis, although it is a more costly imaging procedure than X-rays and ultrasound and is not as widely available. Unlike X-rays, an MRI scan uses a large magnet, radio waves, and a computer to produce images of the body. An MRI can help clinicians evaluate joint damage, especially when it affects the spine, knee, or shoulder. Occasionally doctors order repeat MRIs to track the progression of the disease.

An MRI is a safe procedure for most people, although anyone who has any of the following conditions or factors should talk to his or her doctor before having an MRI: a pacemaker, a cerebral aneurysm clip, pregnancy, a cochlear implant, an IUD, severe lung disease, an implanted insulin pump, implanted nerve stimulators, metal in the eye, shrapnel in the body, implanted spinal rods, gastroesophageal reflux disease (GERD), claustrophobia, inability to lie on back for 30 to 60 minutes, and weight of more than three hundred pounds.

SPOTLIGHT ON RESEARCH

In August 2010, researchers at New York University published a study in which they explained a new way to examine the development of osteoarthritis of the knee in its very early stages. The technique involves examination of sodium ions in cartilage and uses a special MRI technique. The concentration of sodium ions reveals the location of glycosaminogycans (GAGs) in cartilage, and mapping the GAG concentration is necessary for the diagnosis of various diseases, including osteoarthritis. The NYU team developed a new way to isolate sodium ions and thus have introduced a noninvasive way to diagnose osteoarthritis that doctors may soon be using as part of the diagnostic process.

Ultrasonography

Ultrasonography is frequently used to help diagnose rheumatoid arthritis because it is relatively inexpensive, it does not involve radiation, and it is a quick procedure. Instead, ultrasound uses sound waves; as sound passes through the body, it produces echoes, which can identify distance, shape, and size of the objects inside. The echoes are analyzed by a computer in the ultrasound machine, which converts them into moving pictures of the joint, tissue, or organ that is being examined.

As ultrasonography becomes more and more sophisticated, it is becoming increasingly important for the early diagnosis of rheumatoid arthritis. Early stages of the disease mainly affect the synovium, and ultrasound is very effective at detecting synovial inflammation. In addition, high-resolution ultrasound can depict 20 percent more erosions than can X-rays.

Clinicians can use techniques known as power Doppler ultrasonography (PDUS) or quantitative ultrasound (QUS), both of which can be helpful. PDUS is frequently used to detect and monitor inflammatory activity in rheumatoid arthritis, while QUS can be used to detect bone loss in osteoporosis, which may prove to be a good indicator of the early stages of rheumatoid arthritis as well.

DEXA Scans

Your doctor may order a dual energy X-ray absorptiometry, also known as a DEXA scan, to help detect early bone loss in suspected rheumatoid arthritis. If your doctor sees evidence of joint damage on X-rays along with an elevated rheumatoid factor, these are significant predictors for progressive joint destruction.

Blood Tests

If your doctor suspects you have arthritis, he or she will likely take a blood sample to help determine which type of arthritis you have. People who have osteoarthritis usually do not have abnormal blood test results, but those who have rheumatoid and some other types of arthritis frequently have factors or indicators in their blood that can help clinicians make a diagnosis.

Between 70 and 90 percent of people with rheumatoid arthritis have antibodies in their blood called rheumatoid factors, although rheumatoid factor can be found in people who do not have rheumatoid arthritis as well. Generally, people who have rheumatoid arthritis but no rheumatoid factor in their blood are in a less severe stage of the disease.

A newer blood test for identifying rheumatoid arthritis measures levels of antibodies that bind citrulline modified proteins (anti-CCP). This test is more specific than the one for rheumatoid factor because anti-CCP tends to be elevated only in patients who have rheumatoid arthritis or in people who are about to develop it. Therefore, the presence of anti-CCP antibodies can be used to determine who will likely get a more severe form of rheumatoid arthritis in the future.

Yet another blood test that may prove helpful is for cryoglobulins, a type of protein and antibody that is not found in the blood of healthy individuals. Elevated cryoglobulins can indicate a variety of diseases, including rheumatoid arthritis, lupus, and Sjogren's syndrome, among others.

FUTURE TRENDS

It may be possible someday to detect osteoarthritis using a blood sample. Researchers have developed a substance called Klarite that allows clinicians to detect very low levels of hyaluronic acid, which is found in low levels in the synovial fluid of the joints of people who have osteoarthritis.

Tests of the Synovial Fluid

If the diagnosis is unclear or if your doctor suspects an infection may be involved, he or she may take a sample of the synovial fluid from the affected joint using a fine needle. This procedure, called arthrocentesis, serves as both a diagnostic tool and a way to help relieve pain in the joint. If the doctor is not able to remove (aspirate) any fluid from the joint, this indicates that the joint is normal. If, however, there is fluid in the joint, it will be tested for factors that might confirm or rule out osteoarthritis.

If the fluid contains cartilage cells, sulfated glycos-aminoglycan, keratin sulfate, and/or link protein, these are signs of osteoarthritis. If the fluid contains a high white blood cell count, it is a sign of infection, gout, pseudogout, or rheumatoid arthritis. The presence of uric acid crystals in the fluid is a sign of gout.

One side benefit of having fluid aspirated from your joint is that it typically reduces any pain and swelling you've been experiencing in that joint. Another is that some-times aspiration of fluid from an inflamed joint also re-moves any white blood cells that are sources of enzymes that can damage the joint.

Arthroscopy

Arthroscopy is a common procedure doctors use to diag-nose problems in the knee and shoulder, including arthri-tis. In cases of arthritis, it is usually used only when other diagnostic tests, such as X-rays, blood tests, or MRI, are not conclusive.

Arthroscopy is a minor surgical procedure and per-formed on an outpatient basis from a doctor's office, clinic, or hospital. During arthroscopy, your doctor numbs the area of the joint and gives you medication to help you relax during the procedure. Once your joint is numb, the doctor makes several small incisions and inserts an ar-throscope into your joint. The arthroscope allows the cli-nician to view the joint area so he or she can determine what type of damage has occurred. Sometimes a physician will use arthroscopy solely to remove fluid as a way to relieve pain and swelling.

Tests for Inflammation

Any test for inflammation could be helpful in diagnosing rheumatoid arthritis and other inflammatory forms of arthritis but not osteoarthritis. One such test is the erythrocyte sedimentation rate (ESR). This test can provide an indication of the degree of inflammation in the body, but it cannot identify any particular disease, such as rheumatoid arthritis. Specifically, the ESR measures the speed with which red blood cells fall in a test tube. The more inflammation present in the body, the faster the cells fall.

Another test for inflammation is a measurement of C-reactive protein (CRP), which is thought to be a better indicator than the ESR for certain diseases. In people who have rheumatoid arthritis, a high CRP level suggests there is significant inflammation in the body. Doctors can watch a patient's CRP and ESR levels to monitor disease activity as well as keep an eye on how well someone is responding to treatment.

BOTTOM LINE

Getting an accurate diagnose of arthritis is important. A misdiagnosis can mean receiving treatment that is ineffective and perhaps even harmful, because it allows the disease to progress and more joint damage to accumulate. You can help your doctor arrive at an accurate diagnosis if you keep a symptoms diary as described in chapter 3 and work with your health-care provider as he or she goes through the diagnostic process as described in this chapter.

PART II

Take Charge of Your Life with Arthritis

CHAPTER FIVE

Let's Get Physical: Exercise and Movement Therapy

Physical activity is a critical component of self-care for arthritis. You may be thinking, *But I hurt, so how can exercise help? Won't it make my arthritis worse?* Long-term studies have shown that people with osteoarthritis benefit from exercise with improved joint health, balance, range of motion, and strength. Individuals who have rheumatoid arthritis can safely engage in moderately intense weight-bearing exercise. Such exercise helps reduce bone loss and joint damage, and it can be done without increasing pain or disease activity.

But often it is difficult for people with arthritis to become motivated to exercise. That's why the Arthritis Foundation and many hospitals, clinics, fitness centers, community centers, and other facilities offer exercise programs specifically for people who have the disease. This chapter looks at the exercise options for people who have arthritis (e.g., walking programs, water aerobics, range of motion, physical therapy), offers a few exercises people can do at home, and provides some motivational guidelines, including how more and more people are turning to the Internet and social networking to stay motivated.

WHY SHOULD I EXERCISE?

Much has been written about the overall benefits of exercise. When it comes to people who have arthritis, there are some specific advantages to getting off the couch and participating in regular, enjoyable physical activity. The National Institute of Arthritis and Musculoskeletal and Skin Diseases and the American College of Rheumatology point out that exercise can

- Reduce joint stiffness and pain

- Improve muscle strength and tone

- Enhance cardiac fitness and endurance

- Increase flexibility and range of motion

Even if the results of your efforts do not seem obvious to you, regular physical exercise can reduce the consequences of not exercising, such as more joint damage, more bone loss, poorer balance, less coordination, limited range of motion, limited mobility, more severe stiffness, more pain—all contributing to a less desirable quality of life and less ability to participate in activities that you enjoy. The rewards of exercise are not always visible on the outside, but they can make a big difference on the inside.

SPOTLIGHT ON RESEARCH

A study published in March 2010 and conducted in the Netherlands reported that people with hip or knee osteoarthritis who adhere to the recommended home physical therapy exercises and maintain a physically active lifestyle experience more improvement in pain, function, and self-perceived effect. Those who continue an active lifestyle after discharge from physical therapy experience improvement in long-term effectiveness of exercise. In other words, keep on moving!

Five Excuses For Not Exercising

Are any of the excuses listed here the reason why you don't exercise regularly? The first step is the hardest one to take, but with some encouragement, which I offer in this chapter, I hope you will push aside the myths and any anxiety you have about exercising and take that first step today.

- **I don't have time.** This is probably the most common reason given. With a little planning and prioritizing, you may be surprised where you can find time. Can you get up 30 minutes earlier each day? Can you add walking to your daily schedule by parking and walking part of the way to work, walking to a store or for other chores? Simple strengthening or range-of-motion exercises can be done while watching television or even while sitting at a computer. Break up your exercise sessions: perhaps a 15-minute walk before work and another short walk during lunch. Arrange some of your leisure time with family or friends to include physical activity.

• **It's too painful to exercise.** Talk to your healthcare provider or a physical therapist about the types of exercises you can do that will not be painful. Exercises performed in a pool, for example, are non-weight-bearing, because water buoyancy relieves stress on the joints. Many exercises can be modified (a therapist can help) if standing or performing certain movements is too painful.

• **Exercising will make my arthritis worse.** This is a common myth and fear among people who have arthritis and it's easy to understand why you might think it is true, but it's not. The secret is to do appropriate exercise: activity that your health-care provider and/or therapist has determined is best for you and that you enjoy doing. Inappropriate exercise can overwork your joints and result in inflammation and pain, which certainly will not encourage you to want to do more exercise! Even if you are experiencing a flare-up of your arthritis, you can still do gentle range-of-motion or mild stretching exercises. It is important to continue with at least some form of activity when you are experiencing a flare-up, so you will not become complacent and also lose the progress you have made thus far.

• **It costs too much to join a gym or health club.** Gym and health club memberships can be costly, but many offer specials and introductory trials that will at least allow you to see if joining a facility is right for you. But you don't need to belong to an expensive club to exercise. Many cities and towns have community centers, senior centers, and hospital- or clinic-based programs that offer exercise and fitness classes, including those in water aerobics, tai chi, yoga, and other activities. Frequently classes are available especially for people who have arthritis. You can also buy inexpensive equipment (such as hand weights) to work out at home. If you do, don't forget to check out the tips in the "Motivation!" section in this chapter.

• **I tried exercise before and it didn't work.** What do you mean it didn't work? Sometimes people get frustrated with an exercise routine or program and just say, "It's not working." Did you get bored? Was it too painful? Were you unsure about what exercises were safe for you to do? Did you feel like you weren't "doing it right"? Once you can identify the reason why you "failed" at exercise in the past, you can find a solution and start again. It is never too late, and the best time to begin is right now.

Joseph, a 61-year-old sales administrator who was diagnosed with osteoarthritis about five years ago, says he's the "poster child" for exercise and arthritis. "You know all the reasons why people with arthritis say they can't exercise? Well, I knew every one of them, and I would quote them all the time.

"Then one day my wife told me I had better start exercising now, because she didn't want to have to wheel me around in a wheelchair in a few years. She could have been exaggerating a little, but she had a point. I figured I was headed for a hip replacement, and although lots of people get them, the idea of surgery didn't appeal to me. So we bought an exercise bike, and I ride it while watching television nearly every night. My wife and I walk four to five days a week, and she even does stretching exercises with me, so she keeps me motivated. I will admit the pain is much improved and the stiffness is better, too. I feel like I'm one step ahead of a hip replacement, and I'd like to keep it that way."

OKAY, I'LL EXERCISE; NOW WHAT?

Before you start an exercise program, you need to stop and consult your doctor to determine which exercises and other physical activities best suit you and your goals. You may also want to consult a physical or occupational therapist. A physical therapist can show you the proper ways to perform certain types of exercise and the precautions you should take. An occupational therapist can show you how to perform daily activities without placing unnecessary stress or strain on your joints. He or she can also help you with any assistive devices that can make your life easier (see chapter 11 for a discussion of assistive devices).

How much exercise should you do? Your doctor can best answer that question. According to the U.S. Department of Health and Human Services, adults should participate in a minimum of 2 hours and 30 minutes of moderate-intensity aerobic activity each week or 1 hour and 15 minutes of vigorous aerobic physical activity per week. The amount you do may vary, but the important thing is to set goals, keep moving, and stay motivated. I show you how to accomplish all three as I go through this chapter.

MOTIVATION!

Technology is the arthritis patient's friend when it's time to exercise. If you have a buddy to share your exercise sessions with, great! You can motivate each other. However, if you are exercising alone or with your dog, the experience can be more enjoyable and motivating if you plug into a podcast that provides motivating tips and ideas or if you listen to your iPod or another device that plays your favorite music while you exercise. The Arthritis Foundation's program Let's Move Together has a Web site that offers dozens of podcasts (and transcripts online for those who do not have an iPod) on topics ranging from arthritis and golf to indoor biking tips, gardening with arthritis, water exercises, yoga and arthritis, and how to psyche yourself up for exercise.

Perhaps you would prefer to watch—and participate!—rather than listen. The Internet comes in handy here. An Internet search for "arthritis exercise videos" will give you hundreds of sites to visit to either view videos on your computer or learn how you can order or find videos/DVDs for use at home. You can also check your local library's video collection and borrow arthritis exercise videos for free. The Arthritis Foundation has a video, *Take Control with Exercise,* that you can view segments of online or order for yourself.

There is motivation all around you: family, friends, videos, tips, chat rooms, and support groups. Reach out, step up, and step out! You'll be moving and enjoying yourself in no time.

STRETCH, FLEX, RANGE OF MOTION

Have you ever watched a cat stretch? Its movements are slow and deliberate, with every muscle coming alive as the feline stretches and flexes its muscles. Stretching exercises (also called flexibility and range-of-motion exercises) are the most important of all the exercises people who have arthritis can do. If you are having a bad day, your arthritis is flaring up, and you really hurt, gentle stretching can still be done (with your doctor's permission). One wonderful thing about stretching exercises is that they can be done while sitting, standing, lying down, on land or in water.

Individuals with arthritis often have limited range of motion, especially in their hips and knees. Decreased range of motion in these two common types of osteoarthritis is associated with pain, loss of function, physical limitations, and an increased risk of falling. Flexibility exercises can help you get moving. They can improve your range of motion, help you protect your joints by reducing the risk of joint injury, release tension and stress from your body, and help you warm up for more active exercise.

Your joints also need to be fed regularly and well, and when you do stretching and flexibility exercises you provide the nutrition that they need. Range-of-motion exercises compress and decompress the cartilage in the joints, which stimulates repair and remodeling.

Talk to your doctor about the types of range-of-motion exercises that are best for you and how long your sessions should be. Stretching exercises can help ease your stiff joints awake in the morning, and stretching early each day can be the boost that gets you going. If you are not used to exercising, begin with just a few minutes of stretching each day and gradually work up to 15 minutes of flexibility exercises per day. Your doctor can advise you about when you should be ready to add aerobic exercises and strengthening exercises to your program.

Here are a few examples of range-of-motion exercises.

Perform these or similar exercises daily. Gentle stretching and flexibility movements allow your joints to go through their range of motion and can help you reach and maintain flexibility in your joints, reduce pain, and improve functioning.

Many of these exercises can be done just about anywhere: while you are waiting in line at the grocery store, while you watch TV, when you are talking on the phone, when you're at the office. For best results, you may want to do them several times a day: talk to your doctor.

ROM for the Neck

This exercise can be done while sitting or standing, while waiting in line at the bank or grocery store, or even while talking on the phone:

- Gently turn your head to the right, return to the front, and then turn to the left.

- While looking forward, tilt your head toward your left shoulder and then to the right shoulder.

- Repeat these movements 3 to 5 times, 2 or 3 times a day.

ROM for the Fingers

This is another exercise that can be done just about anywhere, including while you are lying down:

- Make a loose fist with your hand; then open it.

- Touch your thumb to each fingertip, one at a time, touching each fingertip twice.

- Spread your fingers wide apart and then bring them together to form a loose fist.

- Repeat with the other hand.

ROM for Your Knees, Hips, and Legs

- Sit in a chair that allows you to keep your back straight and your feet flat on the floor.

- Lift one knee straight up about 3 inches off of the chair, hold it up for 5 seconds, then lower it. Repeat with the other knee.

- From the same seated position, straighten your leg out at the knee, hold for 2 to 3 seconds, then bring your knee back down and rest your foot on the floor. Repeat with the other leg.

- While lying down on your back in bed, move one leg out to the side, parallel to the bed, keeping your knee and leg straight, then bring it back to the center. Repeat with the other leg. Alternate, moving 5 to 6 times to each side.

ROM for Your Ankles

- While sitting, lift your leg and press your foot down at the ankle toward the floor, then bend it back up. Repeat 8 to 10 times with each foot.

- Lift your leg and make circular motions with your ankles, to the right and to the left, one ankle at a time.

ROM for Your Lower Back

- Bend forward at the waist at about 20 degrees.

- Place your hands on your hips and bend to the left, come back to center, then bend to the right. Repeat this sequence 8 to 10 times.

ROM for Your Wrists

- Curl your hand toward your wrist, then move it back the other way as far as is comfortable. Repeat 5 to 6 times with each wrist.

- Make circular motions with each wrist.

ROM for Your Shoulders

- Lie down on a bed on your back and raise your left arm at the shoulder above your head. Keep your elbow straight.

- Stretch your right arm across your body as far as is comfortable.

- Return your right arm to your side and repeat 5 to 6 times.

- Switch and repeat the exercise for the other arm.

DID YOU KNOW?

The Mayo Clinic has a Web site that offers a slide show for people with arthritis on how to do hand exercises. Visit www.mayoclinic.com/health/arthritis/AR00030 or search for "Mayo Clinic arthritis hand exercises."

In addition to the range-of-motion exercise examples, you may also want to consider tai chi and yoga. Both of these gentle practices have been shown scientifically to improve flexibility, balance, muscle strength, and range of motion. Both tai chi and yoga have become so popular in the United States that most towns and cities have community and senior centers that offer classes. Check with your health-care provider or therapist for opportunities in your area.

Tai Chi

Tai chi is a traditional form of gentle exercise that has been practiced for more than six hundred years in China. It is more than a physical activity: it exercises the mind and spirit as well. Tai chi involves slow, flowing, synchronized movements that can help strengthen muscles, increase range of motion and flexibility, improve balance, relax the mind, and boost energy. It requires no special equipment and only that you wear comfortable clothing. Tai chi has become very popular in the United States and is offered at many senior and community centers, as well as some hospitals, clinics, and HMOs.

Numerous studies have been conducted on the effectiveness of tai chi in people with osteoarthritis, especially of the knees and hips. One recent study done by researchers at Tufts University School of Medicine in Boston included 40 patients with an average age of 65 who had knee osteoarthritis. Half of the individuals participated in tai chi sessions for one hour twice a week for 12 weeks, while the other half attended wellness classes and stretching sessions. At the end of the study, those who had participated in tai chi had greater improvements in pain, physical function, depression, self-efficacy, and overall quality of life than those in the control group.

There are several forms of tai chi, and some are more strenuous than others. A modified version of the Sun form has been modified by Dr. Paul Lam, a family physician in Sydney, Australia, and an arthritis patient himself. In 1974 he decided to help others fight arthritis with tai chi, and he began teaching the modified Sun form to potential instructors and the general public. The modified Sun form is especially helpful for people who have never tried tai chi before, as it does not involve any complex movements or strength.

By 2009 more than 1 million people around the world had learned from Dr. Lam's Tai Chi for Health programs. It has been embraced by various arthritis foundations, including the Arthritis Foundation of Australia, Arthritis Care of the UK, and most recently the Arthritis Foundation in the United States, which collaborated with Dr. Lam to produce an instructional DVD, *Tai Chi for Arthritis: 12 Lessons with Dr. Paul Lam*. The course is the basis for the Arthritis Foundation's tai chi program, which is offered at local Arthritis Foundation chapters.

Yoga

Yoga is another practice with Eastern origins that combines mind, body, and spirit, but this one goes back about five thousand years. Regular practice of yoga can strengthen and relax stiff muscles, improve flexibility and balance, provide a sense of calmness and tranquility, and also help with weight loss.

The word "yoga" scares many people because they imagine they will be asked to bend and twist into impossible poses. Not true! First, there are many different types of yoga—Ashtanga, Bikram, Hatha, Iyengar, Kundalini, and about one hundred more—but all of them are based on the same main poses. The differences lie in the pace at which people move from pose to pose, whether a certain type focuses more on breath, meditation, or the physical poses themselves, how long poses are held, and other factors. Hatha yoga is the most popular style in the United States, and it is considered a gentle, slow-moving form that serves as a good introduction to the basic poses and one that people with arthritis typically find the easiest to do and enjoy.

If you want to try something a little different, you might turn to chair yoga. According to an article in *Arthritis Today,* published by the Arthritis Foundation, a growing number of yoga and senior centers are offering chair yoga, which allows participants to practice yoga moves while seated in a chair or wheelchair. Classes can include some standing poses that involve using the chair as a prop to help participants balance as they stretch.

The best way to learn yoga is to attend beginning classes, which are offered by many community centers, senior centers, health and fitness clubs, and even hospitals and clinics. Look for a certified yoga instructor who is used to working with people who have arthritis. For help you can ask your physical therapist or health-care provider for a referral or visit the American Yoga Association, the International Association of Yoga Therapists, or the Yoga Alliance for instructors in your area.

STRENGTHENING EXERCISES

When you have arthritis, having strong muscles can significantly reduce the stress you place on your joints. Regular practice of strengthening exercises can help build your muscles so they can absorb jarring and shock and protect your joints from harm. We are not talking about building bulk, just enough strength to provide protection for your joints.

Strengthening exercises use weights and/or resistance to make your muscles work harder, which then makes them stronger. Isometric exercises are one type of strengthening exercise, and they are especially good for people who have arthritis because it is easy to target the muscles around a joint with these exercises, which reduces stress on the joint and allows you to work the muscles without moving the joint.

Another type of strengthening exercise is isotonic, which strengthens the muscles by moving the joint. One example is the ROM exercise for your leg in which you straighten your leg out at the knee while sitting in a chair. This exercise helps to strengthen the thigh muscle while engaging the joint. Isotonic exercise benefits people with arthritis because you can do a more gentle version when you have an inflamed joint and try a more difficult version by adding weights or more repetitions when you feel better.

To get the most benefit from strengthening exercises, do them every other day after you have done flexibility exercises to warm up. Specific strengthening exercises can be done for different joints, and you should do them only if you are comfortable.

Here are a few examples of strengthening exercises. Your doctor or therapist can help you choose the exercises that are best for your condition. You can see videos of different isometric and isotonic exercises on the Internet on professional Web sites such as that of the University of Washington Department of Orthopedics and Sports Medicine (www.orthop.washington.edu).

For the Chest

- Place the palms of your hands together in front of your chest. Keep your elbows at your sides.

- Press your palms together and hold for a count of 5. Relax for several seconds, then repeat 8 to 10 times.

For the Abdominal Muscles

- Sit in a chair that allows you to press your back against it. Place one hand on your stomach. Inhale, then exhale, and tighten your abdominal muscles as you press your lower back against the chair.

- Hold the press for a count of 5. Relax, breathe normally, then repeat 8 to 10 times.

For the Back

- Lie on your back on a firm but comfortable surface. Bend your knees and place your feet flat on the floor.

- Tighten your buttocks and roll your pelvis up so that you press your upper back against the floor.

- Hold for 5 seconds, then relax. Repeat 5 to 8 times.

AEROBIC EXERCISES

Aerobic exercise, also known as cardiovascular or endurance exercise, includes activities that increase the heart rate and breathing rate for an extended period of time and that engage the large muscles of the body in repetitive, continuous motions. For people who have arthritis, regular participation in aerobic exercise has many benefits, including improved circulation, stronger muscles (which reduces stress on the joints), weight control (which reduces pressure on the joints), better sleep, reduced anxiety and depression, and promotion of overall fitness.

Types of Aerobic Exercise

Topping the list of aerobic exercises that are most effective and safe for people who have arthritis are walking, swimming, and biking (including stationary bikes). Walking is especially easy because you don't need any special equipment (but sturdy walking shoes are a must) and it is much less stressful than jogging or running. Biking places less stress on the foot, ankle, and knee joints, and swimming is ideal because water provides buoyancy and greatly reduces pressure on joints. Many people also enjoy dancing, low-impact aerobics, and yard work such as mowing the grass or raking leaves.

Time to Move!

To enjoy optimal benefits from aerobic exercise, experts generally recommend that you perform your chosen activity continuously for at least 30 minutes. Both before and after your aerobic exercise, include at least 5 to 10 minutes of warm-up with range-of-motion exercises, so an entire session will last about 40 to 50 minutes. If you are thinking, *I don't have time to do that!* you can spread out your exercise into smaller segments throughout the day. Make it your goal to engage in aerobic activity three to four times per week and to work at your target heart rate for 30 minutes each session. (See "What Is Your Target Heart Rate?")

WHAT IS YOUR TARGET HEART RATE?

To calculate your maximum heart rate, subtract your age from 220. Your goal is to exercise at a level of intensity that is 60 to 80 percent of your maximum heart rate. For example, if you are 60, your maximum heart rate is 160 and your target range is 96 to 128 beats per minute.

When you exercise, you should not overexert yourself: aerobic exercise should be done at a steady pace that allows you to speak normally. Be sure to talk to your health-care provider or therapist about what intensity of exercise is most appropriate for your fitness level.

Aerobic Exercise Tips

Water aerobics and water exercise (also called aquatherapy) can be especially helpful for people who have arthritis, not only because the buoyancy of the water removes much of the stress from the joints but also because warm (not hot) water can increase circulation and provide a safe environment in which to exercise. Exercising in hot water should be avoided because of the risk of hyperthermia. If you want to sit in a hot tub as a form of heat therapy, do not stay in the water for more than 10 to 15 minutes and do not exercise in the water.

People who have arthritis should walk as much as possible, even if they must do so slowly, because it offers so many benefits. In addition to being a low-impact activity, walking improves circulation, enhances stamina, reduces fatigue, strengthens bones (and thus reduces the risk of osteoporosis), improves joint flexibility, and strengthens and tones muscles, which reduces the stress placed on joints.

Regular walking is also important because it can help you maintain your independence as you grow older with arthritis. By walking now you can be sure of being able to continue walking well for many years to come. If you get bored when you walk, take along an iPod and listen to music, motivational tapes, or stories. Safety is of utmost importance, so if you live in an area where it is not safe to walk alone find a buddy to walk with or contact a local walking club. Information about walking clubs can be found at the web sites of the Walkablock Club of America, American Volkssport Association, and Webwalking USA Walking Program (see "Resources"). Also check with community and senior centers in your neighborhood for walking programs, as well as mall walking programs.

PHYSICAL AND OCCUPATIONAL THERAPY

You and your doctor may feel that you could benefit from physical and/or occupational therapy. Either one or both can be a part of your movement therapy and help you make the most of your exercise program and your ability to participate in routine activities.

Physical Therapy

Depending on which state you live in and how your health insurance is structured, you may be able to self-refer to a physical therapist or you may need a doctor's referral. Physical therapy generally focuses on a patient's physical and functional abilities and on ways to improve strength, mobility, stamina, posture, and body mechanics. After you are assessed by a physical therapist, he or she will prescribe specific exercises that suit your needs and level of functioning. The therapist will help you learn how to do the exercises properly so you can do them at home. Performing exercises improperly can cause more damage to your joints and muscles, so the assistance of a professional can make all the difference. A physical therapist can also teach you how to use crutches, a walker, or a cane if you need them.

Your physical therapy sessions may or may not also include other therapies, such as hydrotherapy, electrical stimulation, ultrasound, and hot and cold packs. These may be applied before, during, or after exercise, and your therapist can show you how you can use these methods at home as part of your program.

Occupational Therapy

An occupational therapist can show you ways to reduce the stress on your joints during routine daily activities, including how to modify your home and work environments to reduce the amount of movements that might make your arthritis worse. He or she may also recommend assistive devices that may help you with personal care or tasks around the house and show you how to use them.

The Alexander Technique

The Alexander Technique is a painless, noninvasive movement therapy that is sometimes used by physical therapists or by arthritis patients who seek the treatment on their own. This technique can help individuals find improved balance, ease, and freedom of movement in everyday activities, such as standing, walking, and sitting. Alexander Technique teachers retrain people how to move in ways that support rather than harm their joints. Participation in Alexander Technique sessions can improve posture, increase confidence in your ability to move with greater comfort and ease, and help protect your joints. If you have a physical therapist, you can ask about the Alexander Technique and whether it may help you. Teachers can be found through the American Society for the Alexander Technique (see "Resources").

Feldenkrais Method

Similar in some ways to the Alexander Technique, the Feldenkrais Method teaches you patterns of movement that can help relieve your pain, optimize your flexibility, and improve how your body moves overall. The method is taught either in small group sessions known as Awareness Through Movement, where you are shown gentle movements that you can do while you sit, stand, or lie down. You can also choose to have one-on-one consultations, known as Functional Integration, in which the teacher uses his or her hands to guide you through the different movements.

The Feldenkrais Method is very safe and gentle and can be of significant benefit in treating osteoarthritis and rheumatoid arthritis. Much more information about the method, as well as how to find a teacher in your area, can be found at the Feldenkrais Method of Somatic Education Web site (see "Resources").

BOTTOM LINE

Regular physical activity and exercise that are tailored to your needs and abilities and that are enjoyable can help make it possible for you to stay active and independent for many years to come. The benefits of exercise may not always be obvious to you, but if you do not do it, it is very likely you will not be able to remain active and you will experience physical limitations that will adversely affect your quality of life. So be active today so you can stay active tomorrow.

CHAPTER SIX

Treating Arthritis with Medications

At one time or another, most people who have arthritis take medication, whether it is over-the-counter, prescription, or both, oral or topical. Because these drugs typically are used for many years, it is critical to understand the benefits, side effects, and contraindications of these drugs and how they may interact with other medications as well as with foods, supplements, and alternative remedies.

In this chapter I explore these issues for six main categories of drugs used to treat osteoarthritis, rheumatoid arthritis, and gout. The categories are nonsteroidal anti-inflammatory drugs (NSAIDs), analgesics (pain relievers), biologic response modifiers, corticosteroids, disease-modifying antirheumatic drugs (DMARDs), and gout medications.

NONSTEROIDAL ANTI-INFLAMMATORY DRUGS

Nonsteroidal anti-inflammatory drugs (NSAIDs) are the most commonly used medications for the treatment of osteoarthritis, rheumatoid arthritis, and gout. Available both over-the-counter and by prescription, they fight FIP:

fever, inflammation, and pain. They are able to accomplish this through a series of events, which I will explain briefly.

The body produces chemicals called prostaglandins, which promote fever, inflammation, and pain, but on the positive side, they also protect the stomach lining from damaging effects of acid. Prostaglandins are produced by two enzymes, cyclooxygenase 1 and 2 (COX-1, COX-2). Only COX-1, however, produces prostaglandins that protect the stomach. Depending on which type of NSAID you take, it can block both COX-1 and COX-2 enzymes or it may block only COX-2. In either case, the NSAID should relieve your symptoms of inflammation, pain, and fever. The difference, however, is that NSAIDs designed to reduce both COX-1 and COX-2 also reduce the prostaglandins that protect the stomach, which is why these drugs may also cause ulcers and bleeding in the stomach. NSAIDs that block only COX-2 (COX-2 inhibitors) allow the stomach protector COX-1 to do its job. A COX-2 inhibitor will not completely protect your stomach, however (see "Side Effects and Contraindications").

Drugs in the NSAID Class

The NSAID drug class has three subtypes: the classic NSAIDs, salicylates, and COX-2 inhibitors. Every person responds in his or her own way to a specific NSAID, so it is often necessary to try more than one before you find the one that provides the best relief for you.

Classic NSAIDs

Diclofenac potassium (Cataflam)
Diclofenac sodium (Voltaren)
Diclofenac sodium/misoprostal (ARTHROTEC)

Diflunisal (Dolobid)
Etodolac (Lodine)
Fenoprofen calcium (Nalfon)
Flurbiprofen (Ansaid)
Ibuprofen (Advil, Motrin)
Indomethacin (Indocin)
Ketoprofen (Orudis)
Meclofenamate sodium (Meclomen)
Mefenamic acid (Ponstel)
Meloxicam (Mobic)
Nabumetone (Relafen)
Naproxen (Naprosyn)
Oxaprozin (Daypro)
Piroxicam (Feldene)
Sulindac (Clinoril)
Tolmetin (Tolectin)

Salicylates

Aspirin
Choline magnesium trisalicylate (Trilisate)
Magnesium salsalate
Salsalate (Disalcid)

Cox-2 Inhibitors

Celecoxib (Celebrex)
Bextra and VIOXX have been removed from the
    market.

Side Effects and Contraindications

Although they can be quite effective in relieving symptoms of arthritis, NSAIDs are associated with considerable

side effects, some of which can be serious when the drugs are taken for a prolonged time. The most common side effects associated with NSAID use are nausea, stomach irritation, diarrhea, and gas. The esophagus, small intestine, and large intestine may become irritated as well. Stomach bleeding and ulcers are associated with long-term use of NSAIDs, although even short-term use can be a problem in susceptible individuals.

Because NSAIDs are available both over-the-counter and by prescription, some people are prescribed an NSAID by their doctor and forget to mention that they are already taking another NSAID but over-the-counter. Taking two NSAIDs can be harmful, leading to serious adverse effects. More than one hundred thousand Americans are hospitalized each year because of ulcers and gastrointestinal bleeding related to NSAID use, and between fifteen and twenty thousand die. Liver and renal failure are also a possibility. A study published in the *European Journal of Clinical Pharmacology* reported that the risk of drug reactions that can damage the liver and kidneys is six to seven times higher in reported cases of individuals who have used two NSAIDs simultaneously.

When COX-2 inhibitors (celecoxib [Celebrex] is the only one still on the market) were introduced to the market, consumers were told that they posed little risk of gastrointestinal problems. However, COX-2 inhibitors still pose some risk of ulcers and stomach bleeding, although that risk is less than seen with conventional NSAIDs. Long-term use of NSAIDs is the second most common cause of peptic ulcers.

Both COX-2 inhibitors and traditional NSAIDs may also cause cardiovascular side effects. Although the risk is not great, it is worth mentioning, especially for people who are taking other medications and/or who have a heart condition. NSAIDs can raise blood pressure and counteract the effect of some blood pressure medications. They also can hinder the ability of blood vessels to relax and stimulate the growth of smooth muscle cells inside the arteries. These events can contribute to atherosclerosis.

Doctors often recommend that patients who are taking NSAIDs, including a COX-2 inhibitor, also take medication to protect the stomach. Over-the-counter medications such as Prilosec are available, as are several prescription drugs (e.g., NEXIUM, Protonix, Prevacid). Nonpharmaceutical remedies to protect the stomach may include probiotics and licorice (see "Did You Know?" and chapter 7).

If you are taking OTC or prescription NSAIDs, remember the rule of three: take them only as prescribed (tell you doctor about OTCs), take the lowest possible dose that is still effective, and use them for the shortest time possible.

DID YOU KNOW?

Licorice may help protect the stomach damage that can be caused by use of NSAIDs. Look for deglycyrrhizinated licorice (DGL)—licorice that has the chemical glycyrrhizin removed—because this chemical can cause side effects. A suggested dose is 250 to 500 milligrams three times daily, either one hour before or two hours after meals, of DGL licorice.

ANALGESICS (PAIN RELIEVERS)

Analgesic medications differ from anti-inflammatory drugs in that they work to treat pain but have no effect on inflammation. Anti-inflammatory drugs, however, may reduce pain if inflammation is causing the pain.

Pain-relieving medications can work in two ways: they can block the pain signals that travel to the brain from other areas of the body, or they may disrupt how the brain interprets the signals. Arthritis sufferers can choose from two categories of pain relievers: non-narcotics and narcotics.

Non-narcotic Analgesics

Topping the list of non-narcotic pain relievers is acetaminophen, an over-the-counter drug that is considered safe and effective for mild to moderate pain. Acetaminophen does not, however, relieve inflammation.

Narcotic Analgesics

Narcotic pain relievers are often used when pain is moderate to severe. Like acetaminophen, narcotics do not relieve joint inflammation, but unlike non-narcotic analgesics, they can result in dependency, which means you need more and more of the drug to get the same effect. Narcotics can be used along with acetaminophen or NSAIDs to enhance their effectiveness, but only under your doctor's guidance.

Examples of narcotic analgesics include the following:

• Codeine

• Codeine with acetaminophen (Tylenol)

- Hydrocodone and acetaminophen (Lortab, Anexsia)

- Hydromorphone (Dilaudid)

- Meperidine (Demerol)

- Oxycodone

- Oxycodone and acetaminophen (Percocet, Roxicet)

- Propoxyphene (Darvon)

- Propoxyphene and acetaminophen (Darvocet)

These drugs come in various forms, including tablets, syrups, suppositories, and injections. Side effects associated with their use are similar and include dry mouth, drowsiness, dizziness, light-headedness, false sense of well-being, constipation, headache, loss of appetite, restlessness, nightmares, weakness or tiredness, stomach pain, blurry vision, and problems urinating.

Narcotics act on the central nervous system, and so it is very important to tell your doctor about any other medications you are taking before you begin taking narcotics, to avoid possible serious consequences. Although you should tell your doctor about all over-the-counter and prescription medications (and nutritional supplements), the following medications can be especially troublesome: antihistamines, tranquilizers, muscle relaxants, monoamine oxidase (MAO) inhibitors, tricyclic antidepressants, antiseizure medications, sleeping pills, antivirals, and blood thinners.

Topical Pain Relievers

Some topical analgesics can temporarily ease pain when they are rubbed on the skin over the affected joint. These creams, lotions, gels, and sprays are usually used along with other medications and may help reduce your need for other arthritis drugs. The two main types of topical analgesics are capsaicin, which is derived from cayenne peppers; and methyl salicylates, which come from willow bark and are typically combined with menthol.

Topical analgesics can usually be applied several times a day but should not be used on broken, bruised, or irritated skin and should not be covered with bandages. These medications work by stimulating nerve endings and distracting the brain's focus on the pain in the body.

Side effects associated with topical analgesics can include irritation, redness, slight burning, and stinging. Topicals that contain capsaicin are especially associated with a burning sensation, because this active ingredient is derived from chili peppers. However, in most cases the burning dissipates after several applications and pain relief occurs.

Generally, topical analgesics can be used along with other drugs, but do not use them if you are taking blood thinners, such as Coumadin, dicumarol, heparin, or Miradon. If you have dermatitis or eczema, kidney or liver disease, asthma, or glucose-6-phosphate dehydrogenase deficiency (a type of anemia), you should talk to your doctor before using any topical analgesic.

Types of Topical Analgesics

- Local anesthetics (without analgesic compounds added): BENGAY®, CorProfen™, IcyHot®

- Topicals that contain a type of salicylate: Asper-creme®, MYOFLEX®, Sportscreme®; provide pain relief but do not treat inflammation

- Topicals that contain NSAIDs: Emugel, Voltaren®, which can reduce swelling and inflammation as well as treat pain

- Capsaicin: Dolorac®, Zostrix®; reduce the levels of a chemical called substance P, which is involved in transmitting pain signals to the brain

DID YOU KNOW?

Voltaren Gel was the first prescription topical treatment for osteoarthritis approved by the Food and Drug Administration. It is an NSAID in topical form and is mostly used to treat the hands and knees of osteoarthritis patients.

CORTICOSTEROIDS

Corticosteroids, usually referred to simply as "steroids," are potent anti-inflammatory drugs that can help individuals who have rheumatoid arthritis and other inflammatory conditions. These medications, which include cortisone, hydrocortisone, and prednisone, among others (see box next page), mimic the effects of two hormones that are produced by the adrenal glands—cortisone and hydrocortisone. Steroids help control immune function, inflammation, and stress related to illness and injury when they are prescribed in doses that exceed the body's normal levels.

CORTICOSTEROIDS FOR RHEUMATOID ARTHRITIS

Betamethasone (Celestone)
Budesonide (Entocort EC)
Cortisone (Cortone)
Dexamethasone (Decadron)
Hydrocortisone (Cortef)
Methylprednisolone (Medrol)
Prednisolone (Prelone)
Prednisone (Deltasone)
Triamcinolone (Kenalog)

Although steroids can provide significant relief, that relief can come at a price. Steroids, especially oral doses (tablets, capsules, syrups), can cause serious side effects, even within the first few weeks of starting therapy, including increased blood pressure, elevated pressure in the eyes (glaucoma), swelling in the lower legs, mood swings, and weight gain. Longer-term use of oral corticosteroids can cause cataracts, high blood sugar, an increased risk of infections, loss of calcium from bone (leading to osteoporosis), menstrual irregularities, easy bruising, slower wound healing, and suppressed hormone production by the adrenal gland.

Once a patient starts corticosteroid therapy, it can be difficult to discontinue, even at low doses. The usual dose of prednisone is 5 to 10 milligrams daily, although it can be started at higher doses (15 to 20 milligrams daily). However, physicians often attempt to taper the dose over a few weeks to less than 10 milligrams daily. It is important to reduce the dose gradually because some patients are very sensitive to the tapering process and experience side effects.

Because steroids can accelerate osteoporosis, even with a low dose of prednisone of 10 milligrams daily, doctors often recommend that patients undergo bone densitometry (DEXA scan) to determine their risk of fracture and bone loss. Arthritis patients who are taking steroids frequently take bisphosphonates such as alendronate (Fosamax®), risedronate (Actonel®), or others to prevent and/or treat osteoporosis, along with supplements of calcium and vitamin D.

One way to sidestep these problems is to inject the steroid into the affected joint, which targets the drug rather than allowing it to circulate throughout the body. Side effects associated with injected corticosteroids may include pain, infection, loss of skin color, and shrinking of soft tissue. Patients typically can receive no more than four corticosteroid injections per year. Another tactic is to take a combination of drugs in an effort to keep the steroid dose as low as possible. Some patients with rheumatoid arthritis who take steroids take a dose every other day (with their doctor's knowledge) to help minimize side effects.

FUTURE TRENDS

Taking sex hormones could help regenerate cartilage in people who have osteoarthritis. A German team of scientists found that estrogen and testosterone, when injected into the joints, could mitigate the effects of the disease. (Koelling and Miosge, *Arthritis & Rheumatism*, April 30, 2010)

DISEASE-MODIFYING ANTIRHEUMATIC DRUGS

Disease-modifying antirheumatic drugs (DMARDs) are often the first drugs doctors will prescribe for people who have rheumatoid arthritis. That's because these drugs not only relieve arthritis symptoms but also work by interfering with or suppressing the immune system that attacks the joints. Therefore, early, aggressive treatment with DMARDs can help slow down progressive joint damage.

It can take several weeks before you will notice any benefits from taking DMARDs, so doctors often prescribe a faster-working drug, such as an NSAID, an analgesic, or steroids, to provide some relief until the DMARD begins to work. It is also possible to take more than one DMARD at the same time. The DMARDs currently available include azathioprine, cyclophosphamide, cyclosporine, gold, hydroxychloroquine, leflunomide, methotrexate, penicillamine, and sulfasalazine.

Although DMARDs are effective, they also carry a high risk of serious side effects. Therefore, taking other drugs may also help reduce the dose of DMARDs that you need and thus the risk of experiencing any adverse reactions.

Azathioprine

Patients who take azathioprine (Imuran®) may have to wait up to three months before they experience relief from symptoms of rheumatoid arthritis. Azathioprine can cause bone marrow suppression and lower the level of blood cells, especially in patients who have renal insufficiency. Because individuals who have a deficiency of an enzyme called thiopurine methyltransferase can experience azathioprine toxicity, anyone who plans to take this drug should be screened for levels of the enzyme. Side effects of azathioprine can include nausea and hair loss. Patients who take this drug need to undergo periodic blood tests to monitor blood counts and liver function.

Cyclophosphamide

Cyclophosphamide (Cytoxan®) is typically used only for patients who have severe rheumatoid arthritis and who have not responded to other medications. This drug is associated with serious side effects, including bone marrow suppression, premature ovarian failure, infection, and an increased risk of bladder and other cancers.

Cyclosporine

Although you may know this drug as one used to prevent organ rejection after a transplant, cyclosporine (Sandimmune®, Neoral®) is sometimes combined with methotrexate to treat rheumatoid arthritis. Side effects include risk of infection, renal insufficiency, and elevated blood pressure, as well as an increased risk of cancer.

Gold

Gold became a treatment for rheumatoid arthritis by serendipity. A patient who had tuberculosis was getting gold injections as part of his therapy when he noticed that his arthritis was improving. Soon thereafter, gold was introduced as a way to slow progression of rheumatoid arthritis, although it cannot reverse joint deformity.

Gold is effective when it is given intramuscularly. Treatment typically begins with once-a-week treatments and then is tapered gradually over time until dosing is once monthly. Benefits are usually not experienced for at least four months after starting treatments. Gold was more commonly used up until the 1990s, but it has now been largely replaced by methotrexate and other DMARDs. About one-third of patients on gold therapy experience side effects that cause them to stop treatment. Rash is the most common reaction, and it can be severe. Ulcerations of the mouth, tongue, and pharynx can also occur. About 10 percent have proteinuria (protein in the urine). Long-term use of gold can turn the skin bluish, which is irreversible.

Hydroxychloroquine

Hydroxychloroquine (Plaquenil) is an antimalaria drug that doctors began prescribing for arthritis when patients taking the drug for malaria noted that their arthritis symptoms were improving. Exactly how it works to improve rheumatoid arthritis is not known. Hydroxychloroquine is often prescribed for people who cannot tolerate the newer biologics, and it is used along with other DMARDs or with steroids to reduce the amount of steroids needed. Hydroxychloroquine has a limited ability to prevent joint damage when used alone, which is why it is often prescribed along with methotrexate and sulfasalazine.

Hydroxychloroquine is an oral medication that is usually prescribed at 200 milligrams twice or 400 milligrams once daily. Typically it takes two to four months before patients notice benefits from the drug. Hydroxychloroquine may cause low white blood cell counts, nausea, diarrhea, rash, and protein or blood in the urine. High doses can injure the back of the eye, so patients who take this drug should have their eyes checked every 6 to 12 months.

Leflunomide

Leflunomide (Arava®) is similar to methotrexate in terms of effectiveness in treating rheumatoid arthritis, and it can be used along with the other drug in patients who do not have liver problems. Patients who take leflunomide often begin with a loading dose (a greater than normal dose) for several days, followed by a lower dose of 10 to 20 milligrams daily. Benefits become apparent within four to eight weeks.

Patients who take leflunomide should undergo blood tests and liver function tests every two months. Toxicities associated with leflunomide include diarrhea, gastrointestinal upset, hair loss, and elevated liver enzyme levels. Because leflunomide can cause birth defects, it should not be taken by women who could become pregnant or who plan to become pregnant or by their sexual partners.

Methotrexate

Methotrexate is typically the first-line DMARD that doctors prescribe for patients who have rheumatoid arthritis. Why? It works relatively quickly (six to eight weeks), is effective, has side effects that are less severe than those associated with other DMARDs, is low cost, and is easy to take. A comparison of patients who take DMARDs shows that most patients continue to take methotrexate for more than five years, which is longer than other therapies. Methotrexate can reduce the signs and symptoms of rheumatoid arthritis and slow or stop radiographic damage to the joints.

Dosing of methotrexate usually begins at 10 milligrams per week and is gradually increased to a maximum of 25 milligrams per week, although it can go higher. Methotrexate can be taken orally or by subcutaneous injection.

The injection is helpful for patients who experience nausea with an oral dose. Patients who start methotrexate are usually evaluated for renal insufficiency, liver disease, alcohol intake or abuse, low white blood cell counts, low platelet counts, or untreated folate deficiency. NSAIDs are often prescribed along with methotrexate and are considered safe as long as a patient's liver function tests are monitored closely. Methotrexate can also be used along with nearly every other FDA-approved DMARD except leflunomide, which increases liver toxicity.

Patients can enjoy symptom relief as early as four to six weeks, but this response varies among individual patients. If a dosage needs to be adjusted, it may take an additional four to six weeks to determine if the drug is working.

Oral methotrexate can cause nausea or diarrhea, which can be minimized by taking the drug at night or eliminated by getting a subcutaneous injection. Side effects such as mild hair loss, hair thinning, oral ulcers, and gastrointestinal upset may be related to a need for folic acid, which can be improved by taking a supplement (1 milligram daily). Some patients experience headache and fatigue, which can be corrected by increasing the folic acid intake. Serious complications such as cirrhosis, liver damage, and severe myelosuppression (reduction in red blood cell production) are rare, especially with routine monitoring.

Penicillamine

Penicillamine (Cuprimine®, Depen®) is used primarily for patients with aggressive disease who have not responded to other DMARDs. It is relatively toxic and is not as effective as other DMARDs. Major side effects include severe rash and possible damage to the kidneys. Some patients develop a lupus-like or other autoimmune condition when taking penicillamine.

Sulfasalazine

Sulfasalazine (Azulfidine®) is effective overall for rheumatoid arthritis, although somewhat less than is methotrexate. It can be given along with methotrexate and hydroxychloroquine as part of a three-drug approach for people who do not respond adequately to methotrexate alone.

A typical daily dose of sulfasalazine is 2 to 3 grams daily in divided doses. Effects may not be apparent for 6 to 12 weeks after starting treatment. Common side effects include mild gastrointestinal complaints and hypersensitivity and allergic reactions in people who also react to sulfa medications. Individuals who take sulfasalazine should have blood tests every one to three months.

SPOTLIGHT ON RESEARCH

Hydrogen sulfide is a gas that many people associate with a rotten egg smell, but there may be something beneficial and pleasant about this gas as well. A study published in the August 2010 issue of the *Annals of the New York Academy of Sciences* reported that the gas is produced naturally in the body and that it can be found in knee joint synovial fluid. In this study, the investigators found the gas in patients who had rheumatoid arthritis. The good news is that the gas may play a role in reducing inflammation in joints. Now, if researchers can develop a treatment that involves hydrogen sulfide in some way, patients with arthritis may have yet another treatment option at their disposal.

BIOLOGIC RESPONSE MODIFIERS

This class of drugs is approved to treat inflammatory arthritis such as rheumatoid arthritis and works by altering the function of the immune system when it attacks the joints. These medications are among the newest treatments for rheumatoid arthritis and are given by injection or intravenous infusion. The drugs in this category include Cimzia®, Enbrel®, HUMIRA®, Kineret®, Orencia®, REMICADE®, Rituxan®, and SIMPONI®, and they are often used in combination with methotrexate or other DMARDs. Technically, biologic response modifiers, or biologics, are a subgroup of DMARDs, because they slow progression of the disease.

Biologics include several different subcategories as well, which are classified based on how they work. The science behind these drugs is complex. Some target and inhibit tumor necrosis factor–alpha (TNF-alpha), a protein that can cause inflammation and damage to bones, cartilage, and tissue when it is overproduced in the body. Drugs in this subcategory include adalimumab, etanercept, golimumab, and infliximab. Four other biologics, each in its own category, are also explained in this section.

Approximately two-thirds of patients respond favorably to biologics, but these drugs are not without their challenges. Generally, biologic drugs should not be used by people who have a history of recurrent infections, tuberculosis, multiple sclerosis, lymphoma, or congestive heart failure. Biologics are typically associated with an increased risk of infection and should be used with caution.

Certolizumab Pegol (Cimzia®)

Certolizumab pegol is one of the newest drugs approved for treatment of rheumatoid arthritis, getting FDA approval in May 2009 for moderate to severe disease. The drug was originally approved for treatment of Crohn's disease. Thus far it is the only drug in its class, known as a PEGylated anti-TNF medication, and it selectively neutralizes the effects of TNF.

Doctors typically prescribe certolizumab at either 200 milligrams every other week or 400 milligrams once every four weeks. Clinical trials of certolizumab and methotrexate produced better reduction in signs and symptoms of rheumatoid arthritis than methotrexate alone. The drug is administered by subcutaneous injection, which patients can do on their own using a prefilled autoinjection syringe. The most common side effects are upper respiratory tract infections, rash, and urinary tract infections. Serious reactions may include tuberculosis and malignancies, including lymphoma.

Etanercept (Enbrel®)

Etanercept is effective in reducing the signs and symptoms of rheumatoid arthritis and in slowing or stopping radiographic damage to the joints when used alone and along with methotrexate. The most common dose is 50 milligrams taken once per week by subcutaneous injection, which patients can do themselves using an autoinjection system. Some patients are prescribed 25-milligrams doses taken twice per week. It usually takes one to four weeks for obvious results in signs and symptoms to occur, and improvements continue to occur over three to six months.

Etanercept is associated with an increased risk of infection, especially upper respiratory infections. In rare cases lupus has been reported.

Adalimumab (HUMIRA®)

Adalimumab is a TNF-alpha inhibitor that is effective alone and in combination with methotrexate in treating signs and symptoms of rheumatoid arthritis, as well as in slowing or halting progression of the disease. Patients can self-administer the injection every two weeks or weekly, if needed, typically at a dose of 40 milligrams. Benefits of the drug usually take one to four weeks to appear. Side effects are those typically seen with biologics.

Anakinra (Kineret®)

Anakinra can be used alone or along with DMARDs other than TNF-alpha inhibitors for treatment of rheumatoid arthritis. Use of anakinra with TNF-alpha inhibitors may increase the risk of infection. Anakinra works differently from TNF-alpha inhibitors because it blocks the activity of a substance called interleukin-1.

Anakinra requires once-a-day injections, which patients can do using an autoinjection system. It typically takes two to four weeks for symptom relief to begin. Side effects include itching, swelling, and discomfort at the injection site, which affects about two-thirds of patients and lasts for one to two months. The risk of infections, including tuberculosis, is less common with anakinra than with TNF-alpha inhibitors.

Abatacept (Orencia®)

Abatacept is the first member of a class of agents called T-cell costimulatory blockers. Basically, this means that abatacept binds to the surface of a T cell and prevents delivery of signals that can result in inflammation. The drug is administered intravenously once a month after several initial doses are given. Treatment typically takes 30 to 60 minutes, and patients usually see a response within three months. Side effects include increased risk of infection and mild infusion reactions.

Infliximab (REMICADE®)

Infliximab is a TNF-alpha inhibitor that is effective alone in reducing the signs and symptoms of rheumatoid arthritis, but because antibodies can develop against the drug and thus reduce its effectiveness, it is often taken along with methotrexate. One downside of infliximab is that it must be given intravenously and infusions usually take between two and three hours. After the first few infusions, treatment is necessary only every two months for many patients. Benefits from the drug are usually evident within days to weeks.

Infusion of infliximab may cause fever, chills, body aches, and headache. These side effects can be reduced or prevented by slowing the infusion rate or taking acetaminophen, or sometimes corticosteroids before the infusion. Lupus-like conditions have developed in some users of infliximab.

Rituximab (Rituxan®)

Rituximab was originally developed to treat non-Hodgkin's lymphoma. In combination with methotrexate, it is approved for treatment of rheumatoid arthritis in patients who have not responded to TNF-alpha inhibitors. Rituximab works by eliminating B-lymphocyte cells, which play a key role in disrupting the immune system in rheumatoid arthritis. It is given intravenously, and unlike other biologics, the benefits from a single infusion may last up to two years, although it may take up to three months after the infusion to experience results. The initial treatment is typically 1,000 milligrams infused over three to four hours with two doses given two weeks apart.

Side effects may include hives, itching, swelling, difficulty breathing, chills, fever, and fluctuations in blood pressure. Along with the risk of infection, use of rituximab has been associated with multifocal leukoencephalopathy, a severe and potentially fatal brain infection.

Golimumab (SIMPON®)

Another recent addition to the family of biologics is golimumab, a TNF-alpha inhibitor that is approved for moderate to severe rheumatoid arthritis, psoriatic arthritis, and ankylosing spondylitis. In rheumatoid arthritis patients it is intended to be used along with methotrexate. Golimumab is injected under the skin, which patients can do at home. The most common side effects include upper respiratory tract infection, sore throat, and nasal congestion.

GOUT MEDICATIONS

Medications used to treat gout are taken for two purposes: to reduce the severe pain and inflammation associated with acute disease and to prevent an acute attack from recurring, leading to chronic disease. Drugs that fall into the first category include NSAIDs and corticosteroids, which I discussed earlier in this chapter; and colchicines. NSAIDs are generally the preferred treatment for acute gout and are taken for as long as patients experience symptoms. A typical course is to start with a high dose to control the inflammation and then gradually reduce it as symptoms subside.

Corticosteroids can be injected into the affected joint

or a muscle, but they are not as effective as NSAIDs or colchicine. They are usually only used by people who cannot take NSAIDs or colchicine. If you take an oral form of corticosteroids, it is typical to begin with a higher dose and then to taper off within a few weeks.

Colchicine

Colchicine is an effective treatment for gout and has been used for many years. It can be used in two different ways and either to treat an acute attack or to prevent recurring attacks. To treat an acute attack, colchicine therapy must be started within 24 hours of the onset of the attack and can be given every 4 hours. Although this approach is generally beneficial, colchicine is also associated with significant side effects, including nausea, diarrhea, and vomiting.

To help prevent an attack from recurring, colchicine can be given once or twice daily, and then side effects are much less likely to occur. Chronic use of colchicines can reduce attacks of gout, but it cannot stop the accumulation of uric acid that can lead to joint damage even if you have fewer attacks. Colchicine can also be given in combination with probenecid (see "Treating Chronic Gout") on a long-term basis to prevent recurrence of attacks.

Treating Chronic Gout

Two classes of drugs are used for chronic gout: xanthine oxidase inhibitors and uricosuric agents. Xanthine oxidase inhibitors, such as allopurinol, help decrease the amount of uric acid produced by the body. Allopurinol is the main drug used for maintenance therapy in gout patients. Common side effects include headache, diarrhea, rash, and stomach pain. In very rare cases, allopurinol causes a severe reaction leading to liver and kidney failure, and it can be fatal.

Uricosuric agents, such as probenecid and sulfinpyrazone, help the kidneys eliminate the excess uric acid through the urine. While taking uricosuric medications, you need to drink at least two liters of fluid each day to help prevent kidney stones from forming. Probenecid can react with a great number of other medications, so it is critical that you inform all of your health-care providers that you are taking this drug.

In February 2009, the Food and Drug Administration approved the first drug for treatment of gout in more than 40 years. Febuxostat (ULORIC), like allopurinol, reduces the formation of uric acid, and it can be used in patients who have mild to moderate kidney impairment. You should not take febuxostat if you are also using theophylline, 6-mercaptopurine, or azathioprine. Before starting febuxostat, tell your doctor if you have any liver or kidney problems or a history of heart disease or stroke. The most common side effects of febuxostat are liver problems, nausea, flare-ups of gout, joint pain, and rash.

OTHER DRUGS USED FOR ARTHRITIS SYMPTOMS

Occasionally doctors will prescribe chemotherapy for people who have rheumatoid arthritis, because the treatment slows cell reproduction and reduces the levels of certain substances made by these cells that cause inflammation. The doses of chemotherapy used to treat arthritis conditions are lower than those used for cancer treatment.

Antidepressants may also be prescribed if you are suffering from depression. People who have chronic pain such as that of rheumatoid arthritis and osteoarthritis often experience symptoms of depression, yet many do not tell their doctors. I discuss depression and arthritis in chapter 11.

Viscosupplementation

Viscosupplementation involves injecting a solution containing hyaluronic acid into the knee joint affected by osteoarthritis. Hyaluronic acid is not a drug: the body produces hyaluronic acid naturally, and it is found in the synovial (joint) fluid, where it serves to lubricate the joints so they move smoothly and also acts as a shock absorber for stress.

When you have osteoarthritis, however, the concentration of hyaluronic acid tends to be much lower than normal, which compounds the wear and tear of the disease on the knee joints. The Food and Drug Administration approved viscosupplementation in 1997 for treating osteoarthritis of the knee, and it has proved very effective for patients who cannot get relief from painkillers and nonmedical approaches. There are four FDA-approved preparations of hyaluronic acid: HYALGAN, ORTHOVISC, SYNVISC, and SUPARTZ.

Before your physician administers the injection, he or she may remove (aspirate) any excess fluid in your knee. Once the hyaluronic acid is injected, pain relief is not immediate. In fact, you will notice slight swelling, warmth, and some pain at the injection site. If you apply an ice pack, these symptoms will ease. During the first 48 hours after you receive the shot, you should avoid excessive weight bearing on the treated leg, such as jogging, heavy lifting, or standing for long periods.

You may need to receive several injections over several weeks, but the effects typically last for several months.

Hyaluronic acid injections also may stimulate the body to produce more of its own hyaluronic acid. The long-term effects of viscosupplementation are unknown.

BOTTOM LINE

When it comes to medications for arthritis, one thing is certain: there are many from which to choose. Another is that you may be able to reduce your use of medications— even eliminate them—by turning to complementary treatments. That is the subject of the next chapter, where I look at nutritional, herbal, and other natural supplements for arthritis symptoms.

CHAPTER SEVEN

Nutritional, Herbal, and Other Natural Supplements

The most popular form of complementary and alternative medicine (CAM) is the area of nutritional, herbal, and other natural supplements. The number of these supplements available to relieve the symptoms of arthritis is impressive. All you have to do is search the Internet or visit your local nutrition store and you will see scores of products, some providing a single nutrient or herb, lots of combination products, and supplements available as tablets, capsules, powder, teas, liquids, wafers, extracts, and tinctures. Patients give different reasons for trying CAM therapies. First, they have not gotten satisfactory pain relief or improvement in their symptoms from conventional approaches. Second, they either have experienced or are afraid they will experience side effects from arthritis medications, some of which are associated with significant and serious reactions. If you are already taking medications for another condition, adding more drugs introduces the possibility of new or more side effects and drug interactions. Third, they want to complement and/or enhance their conventional treatment with a CAM therapy. Fourth, use of CAM allows them to reduce their dependence on prescription medications. Fifth, they do not like to take medications and want to treat arthritis naturally.

Experts generally recommend that people who want to use CAM therapies do so with the knowledge of their conventional practitioner. This allows for an integrative approach to treatment, one in which all parties are aware of what therapies the patient is taking or engaging in so any potential problems can be avoided. You may be surprised at how good the results can be!

In this chapter I look at the more effective natural supplements for various symptoms of arthritis and the latest research findings on those recently in the news. In the next chapter I cover another area of complementary and alternative medicine: body and mind therapies.

One challenge that faces you as you come face-to-face with these supplements is knowing which ones have been subjected to scientific studies and have been shown to be effective. While anecdotal accounts can be true and accurate and very informative, having validated scientific evidence to back up a supplement's proposed benefits can make you feel more confident that using the product may actually help you, that you are not wasting your money, time, or effort.

HOW TO BUY AND USE SUPPLEMENTS

• Consult your doctor about any supplement you want to take. Make sure he or she knows all supplements you are taking so they can be added to your records.

• Find out if the supplement will interact with other supplements or medication you are taking.

• Know the side effects of the supplement.

- Be suspicious of any unrealistic claims that the supplement's producer may make. It is illegal for the producer to claim that their supplement can "cure" or "prevent" a symptom or condition such as osteoarthritis.

- Make sure you know the safe, proper dosage you should take and how often you should take it.

- Never stop taking any prescription medications unless you have consulted your doctor first.

- Shop around for reputable brands.

- Keep a list of all supplements you are taking and keep it with your list of medications.

- Contact your doctor if you experience any unusual symptoms or you feel worse after taking a supplement. Keep the containers your supplements come in so you can provide information to your doctor if the need arises.

AVOCADO SOYBEAN UNSAPONIFIABLES

Avocado soybean unsaponifiables (ASU) is a natural vegetable extract made from avocado and soybean oils. "Saponification" is a process of making soap from oil and lye. Unsaponifiables are the small amounts of oil that are left over and cannot be made into soap. ASU is a mixture of one part avocado oil unsaponifiable to two parts soybean oil unsaponifiable.

Studies show that this combination of oils has the

ability to slow down the production of some inflammatory chemicals that the body makes, which in turn can inhibit the breakdown of cartilage and promote its repair. A study published in 2007 in *Phytotherapy Research* reported on the findings of 15 studies that used herbal antiinflammatory agents for osteoarthritis. The authors noted that "evidence of effectiveness was strong" for ASU.

In a 2010 study published in *Clinical Rheumatology,* researchers compared ASU (300 milligrams once daily) with chondroitin sulfate (400 milligrams three times daily) in patients with osteoarthritis of the knee for six months. More than 80 percent of patients in both groups reported excellent and good results, and both treatments were well tolerated and safe.

Avocado and soybean unsaponifiables are available in soft gels. A typical dose is 300 milligrams daily. The most common side effect is stomach distress; others include migraine and rash.

BOSWELLIA

You may know this herb as frankincense, guggal, or boswellin, but they are all essentially the same. Boswellia (*Boswellia serrata, B. frereana,* and other species) is gum resin that is derived from the bark of trees from the Boswellia genus, which grow in India. The resin possesses anti-inflammatory properties and is used to treat osteoarthritis, rheumatoid arthritis, and symptoms of bursitis, as well as symptoms of Crohn's disease and ulcerative colitis.

Results of studies of boswellia are mixed. In 2009, a lab study of the anti-inflammatory efficacy of *B. frereana* extracts for osteoarthritis found that boswellia prevented the breakdown of collagen and inhibited the production of pro-inflammatory substances. The authors concluded that *B. frereana* should be studied further as a potential treatment for inflammation associated with arthritis.

In a 2003 study, 333 milligrams of Indian frankincense was given daily for eight weeks to 15 people who had knee osteoarthritis while another 15 patients received a placebo. Individuals who took the frankincense reported less knee pain, better mobility, and being able to walk longer distances than the people who took a placebo.

Very promising evidence comes from Universities of Exeter and Plymouth, which conducted a review of seven studies conducted in humans that examined the effectiveness of *B. serrata* in osteoarthritis, rheumatoid arhthritis, asthma, Crohn's disease, and colitis. The investigators reported that *B. serrata* extracts were effective and that no serious side effects were noted.

A typical dose of the capsule or tablet is three hundred to four hundred milligrams three times daily. Look for products that contain 60 percent boswellic acids, which are the active ingredients.

BROMELAIN

Pineapple (*Ananas comosus*) is the source of this nutritional supplement, which is a mixture of sulfur-containing, protein-digesting enzymes extracted from the stem and juice of the fruit. People in Central and South America have used pineapple for centuries to treat indigestion and to reduce inflammation. Today it is still used for the same purposes, especially to reduce pain and swelling associated with osteoarthritis and rheumatoid arthritis.

Dozens of studies have explored the benefits of bromelain in the treatment of osteoarthritis, and they have yielded mixed results. The first report of its ability to reduce pain and inflammation in osteoarthritis appeared in a study published in 1964. Since then, many of the studies have used combination formulas (e.g., Phlogenzym™, Wobenzym™, and WobenzymN™) that contain bromelain and other enzymes, such as rutin, trypsin, and others. One study suggested that the combination of bromelain, rutoside, and trypsin was as effective as some of the commonly used NSAIDs used to treat osteoarthritis.

Bromelain works as an anti-inflammatory agent by reducing levels of fibrinogen and bradykinin, which results in reduced edema and pain, and by reducing levels of pro-inflammatory prostaglandins.

A typical dose of bromelain is five hundred to two thousand milligrams three times daily between meals. Bromelain may cause stomach upset or diarrhea and should not be taken if you are allergic to pineapples. Because it can increase the effect of blood-thinning medications, consult your doctor before using this supplement. Bromelain may also increase the amount of antibiotics the body absorbs. Do not use bromelain if you are pregnant, have liver or kidney disease, or have high blood pressure.

SPOTLIGHT ON RESEARCH

In a placebo-controlled trial, people with rheumatoid arthritis experienced a significant decline in the levels of pro-inflammatory compounds interleukin-6 and tumor necrosis factor–alpha after taking 100 milligrams of vitamin B_6 for 12 weeks. The study, which appeared in the *European Journal of Clinical Nutrition*, did not show any

changes in another pro-inflammatory marker,
C-reactive protein. The dose in this study was at
the upper tolerable level; the RDA for vitamin B_6 is
1.3 milligrams for adults ages 19 to 50.

CAPSAICIN

Use of capsaicin cream for relief of osteoarthritis and
other types of pain has become more common and is accepted by many conventional physicians as a treatment
option. Capsaicin is the active ingredient in cayenne peppers (*Capsicum annuum*), the red or green, sweet or hot
long peppers seen in many gardens. Medicinal use of
these peppers goes back centuries to the Maya of Central
America, who used cayenne to fight infections, and the
Aztecs, who used the herb to treat toothaches. The herb
has a long tradition of use for arthritis, neuralgia, menstrual cramps, and indigestion.

Modern research has found the scientific reason why
capsaicin has been used by so many people for so many
reasons and for so many years: capsaicin desensitizes the
nerve endings by depleting them of a chemical neurotrans-
mitter that allows pain signals to be sent to the brain. Essentially, the capsaicin overwhelms the nerves, rendering
them unable to transmit pain sensations for a period of
time.

In a double-blind, placebo-controlled study from the
Medical College of Wisconsin, topical capsaicin 0.075
percent was evaluated for the treatment of painful joints in
people who had osteoarthritis or rheumatoid arthritis. The
patients applied the cream four times daily for four weeks.
Capsaicin reduced tenderness and pain in the patients
who had osteoarthritis but not in rheumatoid arthritis as

compared with placebo. Subsequent studies have yielded similar results.

Capsaicin cream, gel, or lotion is available in two potencies: 0.025 percent and 0.075 percent. Patients often start with the 0.025 percent, applying it three to four times daily to the affected area. If this strength does not provide enough relief, you may switch to the 0.075 percent product. Capsaicin often causes some burning and stinging the first few times you use it, but these effects then fade and disappear.

DEVIL'S CLAW

A traditional herb used in South Africa, devil's claw (*Harpagophytum procumbens*) is also known as grapple plant. The plant is three inches across and has wicked-looking projections that resemble claws, but its underground tubers are the source of its herbal remedies, which the indigenous peoples of the Kalahari Desert used for thousands of years to treat all types of pain, fever, and digestive problems. Today devil's claw is used throughout Europe and Canada as a treatment for arthritis.

Scientists have identified and studied several ingredients in devil's claw believed to be responsible for its healing powers. One is harpagoside, and extracts of this substance have proved to have anti-inflammatory and painkilling effects, although not every study has come to the same conclusion.

In a 2002 study, 227 people who had osteoarthritis or low back pain were treated with 60 milligrams daily of devil's claw extract for eight weeks. By the end of the study, 50 to 70 percent of the patients reported improvement in mobility, pain, and flexibility.

In a 2007 study published in *Phytotherapy Research,*

259 patients who had arthritis and other rheumatic conditions were treated with devil's claw in an open study that lasted eight weeks. According to several rating scales, patients had improvements in pain, stiffness, and function and quality of life improved as well. Sixty percent of patients either reduced or stopped taking their pain medication.

In a randomized controlled trial that included people who had osteoarthritis, 45 were given 2,000 milligrams (60 milligrams of harpagoside) devil's claw extract and 44 received a placebo daily for eight weeks. Patients who received the devil's claw reported a significant decrease in pain and significant improvement in mobility.

Devil's claw is available in capsules, tincture, powder, and liquid. The suggested dose is 750 to 1,000 milligrams three times daily. It is best to take between meals, because some studies suggest stomach acid may counteract its benefits. Do not take devil's claw if you are pregnant, have ulcers or gallstones, or are taking an antacid or blood thinner.

GAMMA-LINOLENIC ACID

Gamma-linolenic acid, or GLA, belongs to a group of substances known as omega-6 essential fatty acids. Like omega-3 essential fatty acids, GLAs are necessary for human health, but the body can't make them, which means you must get them through diet or supplements. GLAs are found mostly in plant-based oils, such as corn, canola, sunflower, and olive, and they play an important role in normal growth and development, as well as brain function, bone health, metabolism, and skin and hair growth.

GLA is just one type of omega-6 fatty acid; unlike the others (linoleic acid and arachidonic acid), which promote inflammation, GLA has the ability to reduce it. When GLA is used in supplement form to help reduce inflammation, the sources of the GLA are generally evening primrose oil (*Oenthera biennis*), borage oil (*Borago officinalis*), and black currant seed oil (*Ribes nigrum*).

When you take GLA as a supplement, the body converts it to a substance called DGLA, which is an inflammation fighter. GLA requires some help from magnesium, zinc, and vitamins C, B_3, and B_6 to make the conversion. It can take one to three months before you experience any benefits when taking GLA for arthritis.

Although the evidence supporting the use of GLA to reduce inflammation is not as strong as that for omega-3 fatty acids, it is an option to be considered. A team from Victoria University in Australia reviewed seven studies that looked at borage, black currant, and evening primrose oil for treatment of rheumatoid arthritis and concluded that doses equal to or higher than milligrams per day were beneficial, but doses of approximately 500 milligrams were not.

A study published in the *British Journal of Rheumatology* evaluated patients with rheumatoid arthritis and upper gastrointestinal lesions caused by NSAIDs. For six months, the patients received either 540 milligrams per day of GLA or a placebo. Patients who took GLA showed a significant reduction in morning stiffness at three months.

Black currant seed oil contains 15 to 20 percent GLA, and the typical dosage ranges from 360 to 3,000 milligrams daily. Borage oil contains 20 to 26 percent GLA, and the typical daily dose is 1,300 milligrams. Evening primrose contains 7 to 10 percent GLA, and a typical dose for rheumatoid arthritis is 540 milligrams to 2.8 grams daily in divided doses. Side effects may include occasional headache, abdominal pain, nausea, and loose stools.

A few precautions go along with GLAs. Do not take them if you have a seizure disorder, if you are pregnant (they may harm the fetus), or if you are taking blood-thinning medication. Doses greater than 3,000 milligrams daily may increase inflammation. Some studies suggest omega-6 fatty acids may promote prostate tumor cells, so do not use GLA supplements if you have or are at risk for prostate cancer.

GINGER

For about two thousand years, ginger (*Zingiber officinale*) has been valued in Chinese medicine for its healing powers. Nausea, diarrhea, arthritis, stomach upset, colic, bronchitis, muscle spasms—ginger was called upon to treat them all. Today we still turn to ginger for these ailments, but now we have an idea as to why it works.

Ginger rhizomes (underground stems) contain gingerols and shagaols, chemicals that stimulate the flow of saliva, bile, and gastric secretions, calm the stomach, inhibit nausea, and relieve muscle spasms. There are claims that ginger reduces joint pain and inflammation in people who have osteoarthritis and rheumatoid arthritis and also increases circulation in people with Raynaud's phenomenon.

Study results are mixed regarding the effectiveness of ginger for osteoarthritis. A German study rated it "moderate" for osteoarthritis and low back pain when compared with avocado soybean fraction and devil's claw, which rated higher in effectiveness. A study from Hong Kong used ginger essential oil to massage the knees of elderly patients who had moderate to severe knee pain associated with osteoarthritis. The patients received six massages over a three-week period. When compared with controls (massage without oil and massage with olive oil), the patients who had a ginger oil massage reported significant improvement in stiffness, pain, and physical function at one week after the last treatment, but this benefit was gone by the fourth week after treatment.

A *Journal of Medicinal Food* study published in February 2010 reported that red ginger extract was effective in reducing both acute and long-term inflammation in an animal model, noting that the anthocyanidins, gingerdiols, shagaols, and proanthocyanidins appeared to be responsible for the benefits.

The dried or fresh rhizome is used for supplements. Ginger is available as a powder, extract, tincture, capsule, and oil. The typical dose is up to 2 grams in three divided doses daily or up to 4 cups of tea daily. Because ginger can interfere with medications used for blood thinning, you should not use ginger if you take these drugs. Do not take ginger if you have gallstones.

GLUCOSAMINE AND CHONDROITIN

Glucosamine and chondroitin are often talked about together, because many people take them at the same time, although either one can be used alone. Glucosamine sulfate is a major component of joint cartilage and provides the building blocks for its growth, repair, and maintenance. Among glucosamine sulfate's more important tasks is to help cartilage absorb water and keep the joints lubricated. The supplements are derived from the shells of shellfish such as lobster, crab, and shrimp. Studies indicate that glucosamine is similar to NSAIDs when it comes to reducing symptoms of osteoarthritis, but it can take about one month before you will notice significant benefit.

Chondroitin is a component of human connective tissues found in bone and cartilage. Supplements of chondroitin sulfate are usually made from bovine trachea or pork by-products. Research suggests that chondroitin helps cartilage retain water, enhances the ability of collagen to absorb stress, and blocks the enzymes that cause a breakdown of cartilage. When chondroitin is used along with glucosamine, it may reverse cartilage loss.

Results of studies of both glucosamine and chondroitin are mixed. In a large trial, the National Institutes of Health Glucosamine/Chondroitin Arthritis Intervention Trial (GAIT), 1,583 people who had knee osteoarthritis were given glucosamine, chondroitin, both supplements combined, a placebo, or the NSAID celecoxib for six months. The investigators found that the two supplements together or individually did not reduce pain in patients who had mild pain. However, for patients who had moderate to severe pain, the combination provided significant pain relief when compared with the placebo.

In a second phase of GAIT, investigators evaluated patients who continued to take glucosamine or chondroitin (together or alone) or a placebo to see if they slowed the loss of cartilage in their knees. Patients in all three groups lost less cartilage than expected, even those in the placebo group.

Yet in another study, the results were different. A total of three hundred people who had knee osteoarthritis took either chondroitin alone or a placebo. Those who took chondroitin showed signs that disease progression slowed.

Glucosamine is available in capsules, tablets, powder, and liquid. Generally, 1,500 milligrams daily is the suggested dose, and it can take about one month before symptoms are relieved. Chondroitin is available in capsules, tablets, and powder. A typical dose is 800 mg to 1,200 milligrams daily in two to four divided doses. It usually takes one month for benefits to become apparent. Combination products typically provide 1,500 milligrams of glucosamine and 1,200 milligrams of chondroitin daily.

Glucosamine may cause nausea, heartburn, diarrhea, constipation, and mild stomach upset, as well as increase levels of blood glucose, triglycerides, and cholesterol. If you are allergic to shellfish, look for non-shellfish glucosamine supplements, some of which are made from corn. Side effects of chondroitin may include diarrhea, constipation, and abdominal pain.

Some chondroitin supplements and combination supplements contain high amounts of manganese. Although manganese can help with the production of collagen, amounts greater than the upper tolerable limit (11 milligrams) can result in liver or kidney damage.

MANGANESE

Manganese is a metal and a trace element in the body, which stores approximately 20 milligrams, most in the bones. Researchers have determined that manganese is necessary for proper bone, ligament, and cartilage formation, blood clotting, wound healing, and the metabolism of cholesterol, sugars, and insulin. It is also one of the minerals required to form superoxide dismutase (SOD), a critically important enzyme that protects the body against highly damaging superoxide free radicals.

People who have rheumatoid arthritis tend to have low levels of manganese SOD, which helps to protect the joints from damage. Supplementation of manganese can increase the activity of manganese SOD. Studies suggest that combining manganese with glucosamine and chondroitin can reduce the pain associate with osteoarthritis. In a double-blind, placebo-controlled study of patients who had knee osteoarthritis, those who took manganese ascorbate along with glucosamine and chondroitin got relief from their symptoms.

As I mentioned in the section on glucosamine and chondroitin, manganese is often an ingredient in these supplement products, but you do not want to take too much of it. An excessive amount of manganese can cause loss of appetite, nerve damage, memory loss, hallucinations, elevated blood pressure, and liver damage. Manganese is available as manganese gluconate, manganese sulfate, manganese ascorbate, and manganese amino acid chelates. A safe, effective dosage for manganese is 2 to 5 milligrams daily, and 11 milligrams is the tolerable upper limit. Do not take manganese if you have liver failure.

MSM

Methylsulfonylmethane, better known as MSM, is a naturally occurring sulfur compound found in fresh fruits and vegetables, fish, grains, and milk. Sulfur is necessary to form connective tissue, and it also helps to rid the body of accumulated toxins, which is a risk factor for osteoarthritis. It also seems to act as a painkiller by reducing nerve signals that transmit pain.

Many anecdotal reports and a few scientific studies support the use of MSM for osteoarthritis. In a 2006 double-blind, randomized study, 50 men and women who had knee osteoarthritis were given either 3,000 milligrams of MSM or a placebo twice daily for 12 weeks. Compared with placebo, MSM resulted in significant improvement in pain and physical function impairment, as well as improvement in performing activities of daily living, all without major side effects.

A University of Southampton study in 2008 evaluated

two MSM trials that included 168 patients (52 who took MSM) who had knee osteoarthritis. Reports from both trials gave positive results for use of MSM compared with placebo to treat mild to moderate osteoarthritis of the knee, although the reviewers noted that further studies should be done to identify the optimal dosage and longer-term safety.

MSM is available in powder, tablets, liquid, and capsules and as a topical cream. A typical dose is 1,000 to 3,000 milligrams daily with meals. MSM may cause stomach upset or diarrhea, which can be alleviated by taking it with food. Do not use MSM if you are taking blood thinners.

NIACINAMIDE

Niacinamide is the "other" niacin, a form of vitamin B_3 that shares many of niacin's characteristics but also has some unique ones of its own. The niacin relative is a component of two related coenzymes—nicotinamide adenine dinucleotide (NAD) and nicotinamide adenine dinucleotide phosphate (NADP)—and niacinamide is a critical player in hundreds of enzymatic reactions in the body.

Both niacin and niacinamide have been used traditionally to treat a vitamin deficiency syndrome called pellagra, which occurs among people whose primary food is corn. Today, both forms of B_3 are used for other ailments, and they provide some different reactions at high doses. One of the most obvious differences between the two is that while niacin is associated with the "niacin flush," niacinamide is not. Niacin is used to lower cholesterol and in the treatment and prevention of atherosclerosis, while niacinamide is perhaps best known for effectively relieving symptoms of arthritis.

One way niacinamide achieves this is by inhibiting the activity of interleukin-1 (IL-1), a substance that stimulates the production of nitric oxide, a highly reactive free radical that breaks down cartilage, resulting in osteoarthritis. Research from the University of Toledo, Ohio, also shows that a combination of niacinamide and ibuprofen provides better pain relief than ibuprofen alone.

A suggested dosage of niacinamide is two 500-milligram tablets twice daily or 250 milligrams six times daily for osteoarthritis pain. It takes about four to six weeks before benefits may become apparent. Niacinamide is typically well tolerated and does not cause the severity or degree of side effects associated with the long-term use of NSAIDs, although it can cause stomach upset, nausea, or diarrhea in some users.

OMEGA-3 FATTY ACIDS

Omega-3 essential fatty acids are necessary for human health, but, like omega-6 fatty acids, the body cannot make them, so you need to get them through food or supplements. Cold-water fish, such as salmon, tuna, and halibut, as well as some plants and nut oils are food sources of this important nutrient. Omega-3 fatty acids are also known as polyunsaturated fatty acids (PUFAs), and their tasks in the body include promoting and maintaining brain function and normal growth and development. Use of omega-3s has become popular because they can be helpful in reducing the risk of and treating heart disease, high cholesterol, and diabetes, as well as rheumatoid arthritis, because they have the ability to reduce inflammation.

It is important to have a balance of omega-3 and omega-6 in the diet, yet most Americans consume 10 or more times the amount of omega-6 (found mainly in meats and dairy products) than omega-3 (see chapter 10 on diet). Omega-6 fatty acids promote inflammation (except gamma-linolenic acid; see "Gamma-linolenic Acid" in this chapter), while omega-3s reduce it. Along with adding more omega-3 rich foods to your diet, a supplement can help with symptoms of arthritis.

Several clinical trials have shown that omega-3 fatty acid supplements help reduce symptoms of rheumatoid arthritis, including joint pain and morning stiffness. People with rheumatoid arthritis who also take NSAIDs may also reduce their need for the medication if they take omega-3 supplements. Unlike prescription medications, omega-3s do not appear to slow progression of rheumatoid arthritis; therefore, symptoms may be relieved but joint damage can still occur.

Experts have not yet determined whether omega-3 supplements can help people who have osteoarthritis. Several studies conducted in dogs, however, showed that the essential fatty acid was beneficial both in relieving symptoms and in reducing the need for conventional medication. The results of the studies, which were published in the January and March 2010 issues of the *Journal of the American Veterinary Medicine Association,* involved the use of omega-3 fatty acids administered in the dogs' food.

A few studies have looked at the New Zealand green lipped mussel, which is a source of omega-3 fatty acids, and its ability to reduce joint stiffness and pain, increase grip strength, and improve walking pace in individuals with osteoarthritis. Not all the results were positive, however, as symptoms worsened before they got better for some people.

Omega-3 supplements are typically composed of fish oil capsules that contain both eicosapentaenoic acid (EPA) and docosahexaenoic acid (DHA), the omega-3s found in cold-water fish and in algae and krill. Another form of omega-3 fatty acids, alpha-linolenic acid (ALA), is found in walnuts and walnut oil, flaxseeds, canola oil, soybeans, and pumpkin seeds.

When taking fish oil supplements, base your intake on the amount of EPA and DHA you get, not on the total amount of fish oil. A typical amount of omega-3 fatty acids in fish oil capsules is 180 milligrams of EPA and 120 milligrams of DHA. Five grams of fish oil contains about 170 to 560 milligrams of EPA and 72 to 310 milligrams of DHA.

You may also want to consider krill oil, another source of omega-3 fatty acids. People use krill oil for the same reasons they use fish oil or other omega-3 fatty acids, but krill oil has a few extra benefits. One is that it doesn't cause an aftertaste or "fishy burps" like many fish oil supplements do. Another is that it contains higher amount of an antioxidant called astaxanthin. A study published in the *Journal of the American College of Nutrition* found that 300 milligrams daily of krill oil, when compared with a placebo, was effective at reducing arthritis symptoms and inflammation.

A typical dose of omega-3 fatty acids for arthritis is one that provides at least 30 percent EPA/DHA. If you have rheumatoid arthritis, take up to 2.6 grams of fish oil (1.6 grams of EPA) twice a day. Look for reputable brands that contain fish oils without mercury or other contaminants.

PINE BARK

An extract from the bark of the French maritime pine tree (*Pinus maritima*), which is marketed as Pycnogenol, has shown some promise in relieving symptoms of osteoarthritis. In a placebo-controlled, double-blind study published in *Phytotherapy Research,* investigators enrolled 156 patients who had knee osteoarthritis. For three months, the participants took either 100 milligrams of Pycnogenol or a placebo daily and then were evaluated using several tools. The investigators found that the pine bark extract group experienced a 55 percent improvement in joint pain, reduced their medication use by 58 percent, had a 63 percent improvement in gastrointestinal complications, experienced a 53 percent reduction in stiffness, and improved their physical function scores by 57 percent.

The same investigators conducted a follow-up study to explore the anti-inflammatory and antioxidant properties of Pycnogenol in patients with osteoarthritis who had elevated C-reactive protein (CRP) and plasma–free radical levels. Elevated CRP is associated with disease progression in osteoarthritis. A total of 29 patients were treated with Pycnogenol and 26 served as controls. After three months of treatment, both CRP and plasma–free radical levels declined significantly in the treatment group as compared with controls. These results further supported the findings in the previous study that Pycnogenol is effective for people with osteoarthritis.

A study of one hundred people who had knee osteoarthritis was undertaken at the University of Münster in Germany. The patients were randomly assigned to take either 150 milligrams of pine bark extract or a placebo daily for three months. Patients who took the extract reported significant pain relief, while those on a placebo had no improvement. The benefits of the extract lasted for an additional two weeks after the patients stopped taking it.

No standard dosage for Pycnogenol has been established. The amounts used in the studies of osteoarthritis and rheumatoid arthritis ranged from 100 to 150 milligrams daily. No side effects have been reported.

FUTURE TRENDS?

How about seaweed therapy? Results of a Phase II clinical trial published in March 2010 in *Biologics* reported that a brown seaweed extract that also contained zinc, manganese, and vitamin B_6 provided symptom relief for people with osteo-arthritis, and without side effects. A gift from the ocean may be in your future.

SAM-e

S-adenosyl-L-methionine, or SAM-e, is a naturally occur-ring chemical that is found in every cell in the body and is involved in more than 35 biochemical processes. SAM-e was first introduced as a dietary supplement in 1998 in the United States, and it has been marketed for its anti-inflammatory, pain-relieving, and depression-reducing properties.

Most of the research on SAM-e has been done in Europe, where SAM-e is sold as a drug. In one U.S. study, an Evidence Report Summary, which was sponsored by the U.S. Department of Health and Human Services Agency for Healthcare Research and Quality, a total of 16 medical professionals gathered information from 102 human clinical studies of SAM-e, of which 14 focused on osteoarthritis. After reviewing the evidence, the investi-gators concluded that SAM-e is as effective as NSAIDs for treating the pain of osteoarthritis.

In another U.S. attempt, 61 adults who had knee os-teoarthritis were given either SAM-e or celecoxib in a double-blind study. SAM-e was found to be just as effective as the NSAID, although it took longer for the benefits to occur. Typically it takes up to one week before SAM-e's pain-reducing properties can be appreciated.

A typical dose of SAM-e is 600 to 1,200 milligrams daily. Because SAM-e works closely with folate and vitamins B_6 and B_{12}, it is important that you are getting an adequate amount of these nutrients. If SAM-e is taken at doses higher than recommended, it can cause diarrhea, vomiting, headache, nausea, and flatulence. SAM-e should not be used by anyone who has bipolar disorder or Parkinson's disease.

STINGING NETTLE

Stinging nettle (*Urtica dioica*) is a stalk-like plant that grows in the United States, Canada, and Europe. The plant "stings" because it has fine hairs on its leaves and stems, which contain irritating chemicals that are released when the plant touches a person's skin. These hairs are normally painful, but when they touch an area of the body that is already painful the hairs can reduce pain. Experts theorize that the plant somehow reduces the amount of inflammatory substances in the body and interferes with how the body transmits pain messages.

Herbalists have long used stinging nettle to treat painful muscles and joints, gout, urinary tract conditions, and eczema. Today it is still used for these ailments, as well as for hay fever and insect bites. Thus far, the studies of stinging nettle to treat arthritis have been small and inconclusive, but several have shown that people who take oral supplements of the herb, along with NSAIDs, can reduce their need for NSAIDs. Stinging nettle has high amounts of potassium, magnesium, and calcium, which may make it useful for treating gout.

Stinging nettle is available in capsules and as dried leaf, tablets, tincture, and extract. The suggested dose is up to 1,300 milligrams daily of dried leaf capsules, one cup of tea three times daily, or 1 to 4 milliliters three times daily of the tincture. To make the tea, pour six ounces of boiling water over three or four teaspoons of dried leaves and steep for three to five minutes. Nettle may interfere with blood thinners, heart medications, and antidiabetes drugs and may lower blood pressure.

THUNDER GOD VINE

A vine-like plant from Asia called the thunder god vine (*Tripterygium wilfordii*) has been used by Chinese medicine practitioners for centuries to treat conditions that involve inflammation or a hyperactive immune system. Now scientists have put the root of this vine to the test and discovered that the herb may fight inflammation, suppress the immune system, and have some anticancer effects. The number of tests conducted, however, has been small.

Thunder god vine can be used both orally and topically to treat rheumatoid arthritis. A small study funded by the National Institute of Arthritis and Musculoskeletal and Skin Diseases found that an oral form of the herb may improve symptoms of rheumatoid arthritis in some people. Another small study discovered that applying the herb to the skin can benefit people who have rheumatoid arthritis.

Thunder god vine is a mixed bag. On the one hand, it appears to provide some benefit for people who have rheumatoid arthritis. A typical dose is 30 milligrams daily of the extract. On the other hand, use of the herb is associated with serious side effects, including amenorrhea (lack of menstruation), stomach upset, skin reactions, and temporary infertility in men. This herb should not be used by anyone who is taking immunosuppressive drugs, such as prednisone.

TURMERIC

Do you like curry? If you do, then you're familiar with turmeric (*Curcuma longa*), a member of the ginger family whose roots are used to make the spice that graces so many curry dishes. Curcumin is the active ingredient in turmeric, and it not only gives the spice its peppery taste but possesses antioxidant and anti-inflammatory properties as well.

A closer look at curcumin's anti-inflammatory abilities shows that one way it reduces inflammation is by lowering levels of two inflammatory enzymes, COX-2 and LOX. In a study published in May 2010 in the journal *International Immunopharmacology,* researchers found that curcumin administered to mice with induced arthritis had a reduction in the production of pro-inflammatory substances, including COX-2.

Turmeric is available as capsules containing powder, fluid extract, and tincture. Bromelain (extracted from pineapple) increases the absorption and anti-inflammatory impact of curcumin, so it is often combined with turmeric supplements. When taking turmeric/curcumin alone, the suggested dose is 1 to 3 grams daily of the dried, powdered root or 400 to 600 milligrams three times daily of the standardized powder.

Turmeric and curcumin are safe when taken at the recommended doses. However, if you take large amounts of turmeric for a prolonged time, you may experience upset stomach or, in extreme cases, ulcers. Because turmeric can lower blood sugar levels, talk to your doctor before taking this supplement if you have diabetes. Pregnant women and women who are breast-feeding should not take turmeric or curcumin.

"GOING NATURAL" SUCCESS STORIES

Kyle and Christine have been friends for more than 25 years and have shared many experiences together. When they both developed osteoarthritis around the same time in their late fifties, they discussed how they were going to treat it and decided to try different approaches. Kyle didn't want to experiment, so she started with acetaminophen for the first year or so, while Christine decided to try a natural route, beginning with glucosamine and chondroitin and MSM. The one thing they did agree on was the importance of exercise, so they continued their walking routine, which included about two miles three to four times a week.

When Kyle found that the acetaminophen wasn't working as well as it used to, she increased the dose but worried about the impact on her liver. Christine urged her friend to try a natural remedy. "At least you may be able to reduce your acetaminophen dosage," she said. Kyle agreed and after doing some research decided to try devil's claw while still taking the acetaminophen. After several weeks she reduced her drug dose, and after two months she added MSM and was taking acetaminophen only occasionally.

Both Kyle and Christine have continued taking natural remedies and following their walking program. Christine has added pine bark to her program both for its pain-reducing abilities and because it is a potent antioxidant and signed up herself and Kyle for a tai chi class as well!

BOTTOM LINE

The scientific evidence is here: nutritional and herbal remedies have been shown to relieve symptoms of arthritis. As with conventional medications, certain substances work better for some people than for others. Before you try any of the supplements in this chapter, consult a knowledgeable professional for help in choosing the best dose for your needs.

CHAPTER EIGHT

Other Complementary and Alternative Therapies

Along with nutritional, herbal, and other natural supplements, arthritis patients are increasingly turning to another area of complementary and alternative medicine:
body and mind therapies. If you are among this group of
individuals or if you are thinking about trying an alternative treatment beyond natural supplements, this chapter
can help you sort among those that have been shown to be
beneficial.

The growing demand for CAM therapy for arthritis has
prompted mainstream medical centers and hospitals to
offer programs and treatments that have been shown to be
beneficial. While many of the large institutions, such as
the Mayo Clinics and Johns Hopkins, are providing these
services, so are many small and less-well-known hospitals
and clinics across the United States. Your local hospital,
medical school, Arthritis Foundation chapter, or health-
care provider may help you locate such therapies in your
area.

This chapter explores body and mind CAM therapies
shown to relieve symptoms of arthritis. One or more of
the treatments may be right for you, like they are for Carrie, a 43-year-old software developer who has had rheumatoid arthritis for five years. After starting her treatment

with conventional medications, she gradually tried different CAMs until she found a few that allowed her to significantly reduce her need for medication and also improve her quality of life.

"For me, acupuncture, self-hypnosis, and low-level laser treatments have been a tremendous help," says Carrie. "I learned the self-hypnosis because I have to travel a lot for my job and hypnosis is something I can do anywhere, anytime. I prefer to go to my own acupuncturist and physical therapist for the other treatments when I need them. I really like having so many choices."

WHO IS USING BODY AND MIND THERAPIES?

When we look to see who is using different types of body and mind CAM therapies for arthritis, we find that it depends on the population that we examine. For example, a study funded by the Centers for Disease Control and Prevention (CDC) reported that nearly 50 percent of older adults with osteoarthritis said they had used at least one alternative form of treatment during the 20-week period of the study. Topping the list were massage and chiropractic care.

The results from another study show a different story. Investigators at the University of New Mexico Health Sciences Center explored the use of complementary and alternative medicine among 612 patients who had osteoarthritis, rheumatoid arthritis, or fibromyalgia and who used the university-based primary care clinics. Nearly 50 percent of the participants were Hispanic, and they ranged in age from 18 to 84. Ninety percent of the patients had used alternative treatments for their arthritis at some point, and 69 percent were using at least one alternative therapy at the time they were interviewed. This group of patients differed from those in the CDC study in that 34.1 percent were taking oral supplements (mainly glucosamine and chondroitin), 29.0 percent used mind-body therapies, and 25.1 percent used herbal topical ointments. Other therapies included oral herbal remedies (13.6%), alternative movement therapies (10.6%), special diets (10.1%), and copper jewelry or magnets (9.2%). On average, the patients used at least two alternative treatments for their arthritis.

Then there is a recent study from Weill Cornell Medical College in which P. Efthimiou and M. Kukar reviewed the evidence regarding complementary and alternative therapies for rheumatoid arthritis. In their report, which appears in the journal *Rheumatology International,* they note that the use of CAM by patients with rheumatoid arthritis ranges from 28 percent to 90 percent and that some of the treatments, such as acupuncture, herbal medicine, omega-3 fatty acids, vitamins, and pulsed electromagnetic field, show promise in reducing pain.

ACUPRESSURE

Acupressure is an ancient Chinese healing method that involves applying pressure to specific meridian points to relieve pain. Rather than using needles, as acupuncture does, acupressure involves applying pressure using the fingertips or, occasionally, the elbows, feet, or a blunt instrument. Acupressure is an effective method that patients can do on their own once they know which pressure points to treat, and it can be used along with conventional treatments or alone.

Another advantage of acupressure is that you can do it just about anywhere, anytime, and no one will even know. The pressure point located between the thumb and forefinger, for example, can help reduce pain in arthritis that affects the hands, fingers, elbows, and neck. Other points include the point directly below the knee, one between the big and second toes, and another between the fourth and last toes. You can experience pain relief in the legs and feet when applying pressure to these latter points.

You can ask an acupressure therapist or other knowledgeable health-care practitioner who is familiar with acupressure about which points to work. Charts of acupressure points for arthritis are also available online and in books. A Web site called AcupressureOnline.org (see "Resources") provides illustrations of pressure points for arthritis and other ailments.

To do acupressure, here are a few tips. You can also have someone else apply acupressure for you.

- If possible, get into a comfortable seated or lying-down position so you can relax. However, if you are at work, standing in line at the bank, or stuck in traffic and you want to treat a pressure point, that's fine, too.

- Apply deep, firm pressure to each point. If it hurts too much, back off a bit until you reach a comfortable pain level.

- Massage each point and increase the pressure as the initial painful sensation begins to go away.

- Massage each point until you experience a numbing feeling.

- Acupressure can be done as many times a day as you desire.

ACUPUNCTURE

For about two thousand years, the medical art of acupuncture has been used to treat a variety of ailments, but it has not had an easy time entering mainstream medicine. In recent years, however, there have been many scientific studies showing that acupuncture can be effective, and a growing number of physicians now recommend treatments for certain conditions. Osteoarthritis and rheumatoid arthritis are two of them.

Acupuncture is an ancient Chinese medicine practice that is based on the theory that life energy called qi flows through the body along 20 invisible pathways called meridians. According to Chinese medicine, when qi is blocked or out of balance, pain, illness, or disease is the result. There are more than two thousand acupuncture points—the same ones used in acupressure—along the meridians, so it takes a professional acupuncture therapist to know which ones to treat.

Acupuncture relieves the pain of osteoarthritis and rheumatoid arthritis, but exactly how it does so has not been clearly defined, although experts have several theories. One is that the acupuncture needle helps release shortened muscles and allows them to relax; another is that it stimulates the release of endorphins, the body's natural painkilling substances. Acupuncture may also change the brain's perception of pain. Researchers have used magnetic resonance imaging to study patients while they are being treated with acupuncture and found that deep needling deactivates the part of the brain that is involved with pain perception.

One person who had her doubts about the effectiveness of acupuncture is Helen, whose grandmother suffers with rheumatoid arthritis. Helen listened as her grandmother complained that the painkillers her doctor had given her were not working. "My grandmother is from the old country, an Italian immigrant who believes in old-fashioned cures," explains Helen. "A friend of mine is a believer in acupuncture, and she convinced my grandmother to try it. Because it didn't involve drugs, she was willing to try it. After just a few sessions, my grandmother said she felt one hundred percent better. She still goes for occasional treatments, and she's happy with the results."

A type of acupuncture called electro-acupuncture is also used to treat arthritis. A group of patients with knee osteoarthritis reported significant pain relief after being treated with this form of therapy. In electro-acupuncture, the needles are equipped with clips that are attached to a device that delivers a continuous mild electrical impulse to stimulate each acupuncture point. Scientists believe that electro-acupuncture increases endorphin levels while lowering the levels of cortisol, a hormone that tends to increase during physical or mental stress.

In a large German study, 304,674 patients who had knee osteoarthritis participated in 15 sessions of acupuncture along with their usual medical care or just routine care. Those who were treated with acupuncture reported less pain and stiffness, improved function, and better quality of life than the patients who did not undergo acupuncture. The benefits of acupuncture lasted for at least an additional three months after acupuncture treatments stopped.

One of the newest studies of acupuncture in osteo-arthritis patients found little to no difference between "real" acupuncture and fake or "sham" treatments. The study was conducted by investigators at MD Anderson Cancer Center, who included 455 patients with knee osteoarthritis in their study, along with 72 healthy controls. The arthritis patients received either traditional Chinese acupuncture or sham acupuncture treatments that were delivered by acupuncturists trained to interact with their patients in one of two ways: a positive approach ("I've had lots of success treating knee pain") or a neutral one ("It may or may not work for you"). The researchers found no statistically significant differences in symptom relief between patients in either acupuncture group. However, they did see a small but significant effect on pain and satisfaction with treatment depending on the acupuncturist's style: patients who had a provider with a positive attitude experienced greater satisfaction and pain improvement than those who had neutral practitioners. This suggests that a placebo effect may be involved with acupuncture treatment for osteoarthritis.

Some private health insurers cover acupuncture treatments, although Medicare does not. If you need help finding a certified acupuncturist, you can contact the National Certification Commission for Acupuncture and Oriental Medicine and the American Academy of Medical Acupuncture (see "Resources").

APITHERAPY

If "ouch" is the first thing that comes to mind when you hear about apitherapy, also known as bee sting therapy, you are not alone. Yet there are many proponents of bee therapy, who say the sting is worth the relief that it brings for people who have arthritis, lupus, and multiple sclerosis, among other ailments.

Apitherapy is a traditional folk remedy that has been used for centuries in many countries. Modern analysis of bee venom shows that it contains about 40 different healing substances, including melittin, which was reported in at least one study to have anti-inflammatory and anti-arthritic properties. Although few studies have been conducted in people with arthritis, there are several animal studies in which bee venom successfully reduced inflammation and pain associated with arthritis.

A 2007 study performed in China, however, included 100 people who had rheumatoid arthritis. Fifty were treated with medication (methotrexate, sulfasalazine, meloxicam) and 50 were given medication plus bee sting treatment. Treatments were given once every other day for three months. At the end of the study, the patients in the medication plus bee sting group scored significantly better on joint swelling, pain, number of joints swollen, and morning stiffness than those in the medication-only group. Although this study did not show how effective bee sting therapy is on its own, it does show that bee sting therapy can reduce the need for medication among people with rheumatoid arthritis.

It's been reported that about sixty-five thousand people in the United States use bee sting therapy. Many people in the medical establishment say it is not a viable form of treatment and that it can be deadly. Approximately 2 percent of Americans are allergic to bee stings, and epinephrine should always be immediately available whenever someone receives bee venom treatment just in case he or she has a reaction, including anaphylactic shock.

You can get more information about apitherapy from the American Apitherapy Society. However, because apitherapy is not an approved form of treatment in the United States, there is no official list of apitherapists.

DID YOU KNOW?

If you are seriously considering apitherapy, you should undergo allergy testing to make sure you are not allergic to bee stings. Although the percentage of people believed to be allergic to bee venom is low (about 2 percent, although some say as high as 5 percent), you may be one of them.

AROMATHERAPY

Can aromatherapy really help people who have arthritis? Several studies conducted at well-known medical centers say it can. Mehmet Oz, M.D., professor of surgery at Columbia University Medical Center in New York City, says that aromatherapy is effective because the essential oils work directly on the brain's emotional center, the amygdala. Dr. Oz's work with aromatherapy led him to recommend using essential oils, such as lavender, eucalyptus, or chamomile, and diluting them with a neutral oil, such as avocado, almond, or jojoba. The typical formula is 15 drops of essential oil mixed with one ounce (two tablespoons) of neutral oil, which you then rub into your skin. Alan Hirsch, M.D., a neurologist at the Smell & Taste Treatment and Research Foundation in Chicago, points out that people should limit how long they are exposed to certain scents because they will stop responding to the scents after a few minutes. Essential oils associated with benefits include vanilla (lowers heart rate and blood pressure) and green apple (reduces joint pain and muscle contractions).

CHIROPRACTIC

Chiropractic care is based on the concept that the body has the ability to heal itself. A chiropractor uses hands-on adjustments and manipulations to correct joint and spine misalignments and relieve pressure on nerves caused by such abnormalities. Chiropractic treatments can increase the range of motion of the body, which helps the patient move better and with less stress and strain on the joints and muscles.

Approximately 11 percent of Americans had received chiropractic care within the last 12 months, according to the 2007 National Health Interview Survey (latest available data), which translates into more than 18 million adults and 2 million children. Naturally, not all of these individuals were seeking treatments for arthritis, but chiropractic care is one of the more common complementary therapies for the disease.

When chiropractic sessions are a regular part of a person's lifestyle they may help to prevent arthritis, but most people who choose chiropractic care do so after they have the disease. Depending on the extent of your pain, range of motion, stiffness, and other arthritis-related symptoms, regular chiropractic sessions can help reduce fluid accumulation in the joints, improve range of motion, ease pain, and reduce stiffness.

During your initial visit with a chiropractor, he or she will take a personal health history and perform a physical examination, with special focus on the spine. X-rays may also be performed. If the chiropractor believes chiropractic treatment will be helpful, he or she will develop a treatment plan.

Some chiropractors practice only spinal manipulation, while others also incorporate nutritional counseling, dietary supplements, massage, ice and heat, and electrical stimulation as part of their treatments. Spinal manipulation is not recommended if you have rheumatoid arthritis or arthritis of the neck. You should have a cervical X-ray before you undergo any type of spinal manipulation.

Talk to your doctor and physical therapist about whether chiropractic treatments are right for you. You can get more information about chiropractic care and where to find a licensed practitioner in your area by contacting the American Chiropractic Association (see "Resources").

HYPNOSIS

"You are getting very sleepy." That's what some people think of when they hear the word "hypnosis" or "hypnotherapy," but hypnosis is much more than a stage show. Scores of studies show that hypnotherapy, whether it is conducted by a trained hypnotherapist or an individual who has learned self-hypnosis (typically from a professional), is an effective treatment for a variety of health conditions ranging from chronic pain to depression.

Take a Texas A&M University College of Medicine study, in which the researchers reviewed 13 studies that explored the use of hypnosis for the treatment of chronic pain. They found that hypnosis was more effective than nonhypnotic treatment approaches such as physical therapy and education and that self-hypnosis was the most used form of hypnotherapy in the studies. At the Mount Sinai School of Medicine in New York, an analysis of 18 studies of hypnosis and its impact on different types of pain conducted with more than nine hundred people found that 75 percent of the participants experienced substantial pain relief.

According to Guy Montgomery, Ph.D., a behavioral scientist at the Mount Sinai School of Medicine who has done much research on hypnosis and pain, "most patients benefit from the use of hypnotic suggestion for pain relief." That means you could, too. With the help of a professional hypnotherapist, you could learn how to reduce your arthritis pain using self-hypnosis after just a few sessions. All hypnosis is self-hypnosis, because the role of the hypnotherapist is to guide you on the self-propelled journey of applied imagination. Hypnosis is a way to focus your imagination and attention to help reduce physical and emotional challenges. Studies of brain imaging of people who are hypnotized show that some hypnotic suggestions reduce activity in areas of the brain associated with emotional responses to pain, while other suggestions impact areas involved with the physical sensations of pain.

Why does hypnosis work? There are several theories, one of which is that hypnosis changes what you expect pain to be, while another is that when you focus your attention on something outside of yourself your perception of pain is blocked.

Whatever the reasons may be, hypnosis usually helps relieve within 4 to 10 sessions, although some people respond even faster and a small percentage do not respond at all. If you would like to discover how hypnosis may work for you, ask for a referral from your physician or contact an organization that focuses on hypnotherapy for information and suggestions.

LOW-LEVEL LASER

Low-level laser therapy, also referred to as cold laser therapy or biostimulation therapy, is a painless procedure that uses low-energy lasers or light-emitting diodes to stimulate or inhibit the function of cells. People who have rheumatoid arthritis, neck pain, sports-related pain, and chronic joint disorders have benefited from this treatment approach.

Experts are not sure exactly how low-level laser therapy works, although it appears to be effective at only specific wavelengths of laser. People who are treated with laser therapy below the dose range do not receive any relief. Some researchers say the treatments work because they reduce the levels of factors associated with inflammation, such as prostaglandins and tumor necrosis factor–alpha, as well as bleeding and swelling. Another possibility is that laser stimulates the cells to produce the energy molecules called adenosine triphosphate, which, through a complex process, have a positive impact on the cells and reduce pain.

In a review of 13 trials of low-level laser therapy for treatment of patients with rheumatoid arthritis or osteoarthritis, 212 patients received laser treatment, 174 had placebo laser, and 68 received laser on one hand and placebo on the opposite hand. The length of treatment spanned 4 to 10 weeks.

The patients who had rheumatoid arthritis experienced a 70 percent reduction in pain when compared with placebo patients and reduced morning stiffness by 27.5 minutes. The individuals who had their hands treated did not notice a difference in pain relief between the laser treatment and placebo. Of the 197 patients who had osteoarthritis, low-level laser had no effect on pain, joint tenderness, joint mobility, or strength.

So, if you have rheumatoid arthritis and are looking for drug-free, short-term relief of pain and morning stiffness, low-level laser therapy may be a good choice for you. This therapy is offered by pain clinics, physical therapists, sports medicine clinics, and some physicians.

MEDITATION

Although there are dozens of different ways to meditate, all of them have one thing in common: they all focus on

quieting a busy, active mind. According to Joan Bory-
senko, Ph.D., who is a pioneer in the field of mind/body
medicine, "Meditation helps to keep us from identifying with the 'movies of the mind.'" When we are able to
calm our mind and stay focused in the present, the mind
and body respond in positive ways, from lowering blood
pressure and heart rate to reducing depression and stress
hormone levels.

Generally there are two basic approaches to meditation: mindfulness and concentration. With mindfulness
meditation, the intent is to be an impartial observer of
everything that passes by your attention. Rather than
focus on one thought, object, or action, you are to be mind-
ful, fully aware of what is going on in the present moment.
Some people say it's like watching a parade: watching the
action go by without participating in it.

Concentration involves focusing your attention on a
single object, sound, or the breath. This approach gives
your mind something consistent to focus on.

Decades of research have shown that meditation can
help relieve symptoms associated with arthritis, including
pain, inflammation, depression, fatigue, stress, and anxiety. At the University of Maryland School of Medicine,
for example, researchers evaluated the effectiveness of a
mindfulness meditation program on disease activity, depressive symptoms, and state of mind in 63 patients who
had rheumatoid arthritis. Participants were assigned to
either an eight-week course and four-month maintenance
program on mindfulness meditation or a wait-list control
group, who were promised free access to the meditation
program once the study was finished.

At the end of the six-month study, the patients in the
meditation group reported a significant improvement in
psychological distress, well-being, and depressive symp-

toms, although the practice of meditation did not improve their arthritis symptoms. The study's authors concluded that mindfulness meditation may be a good complement to medical management of rheumatoid arthritis.

In another study, patients with rheumatoid arthritis had a somewhat different response to meditation. When compared with patients who received either education only, those who participated in cognitive behavioral therapy or mindfulness meditation had more improvement in coping skills. Patients with recurrent depression got the most benefit from meditation overall, including improvement in joint tenderness.

Mindfulness meditation can be an effective addition to your treatment program. With daily practice, you will soon be rewarded with both physical and emotional benefits.

Mindfulness Meditation Practice

• Find a quiet, comfortable place where you can meditate without being disturbed. You may choose a chair that allows you to keep your head, neck, and back straight, or you can sit on the floor.

• Close your eyes and empty your mind of all thoughts of the past and future. Stay in the moment.

• Become aware of your breathing by focusing on what it feels like as the air moves in and out of your body. Notice how each breath is different.

• Whenever a thought enters your mind, observe it as you would a cloud in the sky, letting it drift by without making any attempt to judge it, worry about it, or ignore it. Just let it be a cloud. Remain calm and use your breathing as your focal point.

• If a thought tries to "take over" your mind, remain calm and simply return your focus to your breathing. Do not judge the fact that you may have been carried away by a thought. Just let it drift away.

• After an amount of time you find comfortable (say, 10 to 15 minutes), sit quietly for a minute or two as you gradually become aware of where you are and then return to your day.

NEUROMUSCULAR ELECTRICAL STIMULATION

Neuromuscular electrical stimulation (NMES) is a form of therapy in which mild electrical stimulation is applied to selected muscle tissue to strengthen the muscle that supports a joint and to relieve pain in and around the joint. If you are suffering with knee osteoarthritis, this therapy may be of interest to you, because several studies have shown it can be quite effective in reducing pain and strengthening the quadriceps muscles that support the knee.

For example, a study published in *Clinical Rheumatology* reported on 50 women who had osteoarthritis of the knee. The researchers found that when it came to relieving pain and stiffness, as well as improving walking time and the ability to use the stairs, a four-week program of electrical stimulation was just as effective as a four-week exercise program. This finding means NMES can be a useful option for people with knee osteoarthritis who are unable to exercise and can actually help strengthen their muscles so they will be able to exercise.

Neuromuscular electrical stimulation may provide another benefit: it can postpone the need for total knee replacement surgery by several years. This benefit was seen in a clinical study conducted at 23 centers across the United States. The multicenter study included 109 women and 48 men who ranged in age from 31 to 88. All had moderate to severe knee osteoarthritis. The 157 patients wore an electrical stimulation device for 6 to 10 hours daily (usually while sleeping), while a control group of 101 patients did not use the device. Sixty-two percent of the patients who received electrical stimulation were able to postpone knee replacement surgery for four years, while only 7 percent in the control group were able to do the same.

One of the benefits of this treatment approach is that you can wear the device at home, which gives you control over the process. If neuromuscular electrical stimulation sounds like something you want to try, consult with your physician or physical therapist or a chronic pain clinic.

PROLOTHERAPY

Prolotherapy, a natural technique that stimulates the body to repair and heal itself, is considered an alternative to arthroscopy, cortisone shots, chronic use of NSAIDs and/or narcotic pain medications, and surgery for people who are having difficulty getting relief from arthritis pain. Advocates of prolotherapy believe these other treatment options, which often are not effective, may also disrupt or even prevent the healing process.

Prolotherapy involves the injection of a substance (a mild proliferant) into the affected tendons or ligaments, which leads to local inflammation. While this may not sound like a positive reaction, it is: the localized inflammation triggers a cascade of healing, beginning with the stimulation of cells called fibroblasts. These are the cells that make new collagen, the substance that tendons and ligaments are made of. New collagen shrinks over time, and this tightens the ligament or tendon and makes it stronger. The secret to effective prolotherapy treatment is injecting enough of the solution into the affected area. Prolotherapy has proved effective in relieving pain associated with arthritis, sports injuries, low back pain, and other conditions.

When we look for studies of prolotherapy that have focused on arthritis, there are only a few, but the findings were positive. Results of two randomized, controlled studies support the use of 10 percent dextrose prolotherapy for osteoarthritis that affected the fingers, while another two studies involving osteoarthritis of the knees also reported improvements.

Prolotherapy is administered by M.D.s and D.O.s, most often those who specialize in orthopedics, physical medicine, or rehabilitation. If your physician or local hospital cannot provide references, you can always contact the American Osteopathic Association of Prolotherapy Integrative Pain Management or the American Association of Orthopaedic Medicine (see "Resources").

POPULAR BUT QUESTIONABLE

Several popular alternative treatments for arthritis may be used by a significant number of people, but scientific evidence to support their use is largely lacking. Here are a few of the therapies that fall into the category "Popular but Questionable."

Copper Bracelets

The situation regarding the use of copper bracelets and other copper objects for arthritis relief is similar to that for magnet therapy: no scientific evidence, no adverse effects, and the possibility of placebo effect and hope. One popular theory about why copper bracelets work is that copper salts, which have antioxidant properties, penetrate the skin from the bracelet or other copper jewelry and attack free radicals. However, skin is unable to absorb the amount of copper salts it would take to prevent free-radical damage.

Magnet Therapy

Magnets produce a force called a magnetic field, and the strength of the field is measured in units called gauss (G). Magnets sold to relieve pain usually claim to have strengths ranging from 300 to 5,000 G, which is much stronger than the Earth's magnetic field but weaker than the magnets found in MRI machines. Magnet products marketed for health purposes include shoe insoles, bracelets, mattress pads, headbands, belts, and bandages. Thus far, there has not been any scientific evidence that magnets help relieve pain, inflammation, or stiffness associated with osteoarthritis or rheumatoid arthritis. The best that can be said about magnet therapy is that it does not seem to cause any adverse effects and it offers hope to some people. Anecdotal success stories may be demonstrations of the placebo effect.

BOTTOM LINE

Every day, people who have arthritis are turning to the alternative and complementary therapies discussed in this chapter to treat symptoms of arthritis. We hope one or more of them open a door of opportunity and relief for you or a loved one who is living with this disease.

CHAPTER NINE

Surgical Options

Sometimes over-the-counter and prescription drugs, medical procedures, nutritional therapy, and complementary treatments just are not enough to provide sufficient relief from the pain and other symptoms of arthritis. It may be that your quality of life is just not what you want it to be or what you deserve, or that your condition will continue to deteriorate if you do not take more dramatic steps. That's when it's time to consider surgical options.

Surgical procedures to correct and eliminate the pain and other symptoms of osteoarthritis, rheumatoid arthritis, and gout have made great strides over the decades. In this chapter I explore the surgical options available to you so you can be more informed when you approach your health-care provider about your choices. I also look at what to expect after surgery in terms of recovery time, realistic expectations of improvement, and possible side effects and complications.

SURGERY FOR ARTHRITIS

Although surgery is typically the last option most people want to turn to in order to get relief from their arthritis pain and other symptoms, for some people it is the only logical choice that remains. The good news is that there are numerous options from which to choose. Joint replacement surgery, for example, has become one of the most effective treatments available. People with arthritis frequently turn to hip or knee joint replacement, but surgeons are also replacing ankles, shoulders, elbows, and knuckles. Hip resurfacing is an alternative to total hip replacement. Other procedures I will discuss in this chapter include arthrodesis, osteotomy, resection, synovectomy, and washing out. All of these are options for people who have arthritis that is not responding to other therapies.

Are You a Surgical Candidate?

You've been patient; you've tried different medications, medical procedures, injections, and alternative therapies, but you still experience pain in one or more joints and have limited mobility and your quality of life is declining. How do you know if you are a good candidate for surgery?

All of the reasons just stated may make you a suitable candidate for surgery. Other important factors to consider include your reasons for wanting surgery, your current state of overall health, and, to the best of your doctor's knowledge, what your prognosis is. The decision to undergo a surgical procedure is one that you need to discuss with your doctor and a surgeon and perhaps other individuals as well, including other health professionals and family members. All of the people involved in the decision-making process need to be aware of the risks and benefits of the procedure you are considering.

Who Performs Arthritis Surgery?

Surgery for arthritis is a specialized branch of orthopedic surgery that includes professionals known as orthopedic surgeons or orthopedists. Many orthopedic surgeons specialize in specific procedures, such as joint replacement, hand surgery, or sports injuries. You will want to consult an orthopedic surgeon who has done many of the procedure you are choosing, which include those discussed here. For help choosing an orthopedic surgeon, see chapter 3.

TYPES OF SURGICAL PROCEDURES

An orthopedic surgeon may perform any of the following surgical procedures. Many surgeons specialize in one type of surgery, so you will want to make sure your surgeon specializes in the procedure you have chosen.

Arthrodesis

Arthrodesis, also known as bone or joint fusion surgery, is performed to relieve arthritis pain in the hips, ankles, wrists, fingers, thumbs, or spine. The procedure involves fusing each end of two bones together, which eliminates the joint. Arthrodesis is performed for patients whose joints have been destroyed by osteoarthritis, rheumatoid arthritis, or other forms of arthritis. Although a fused joint loses its flexibility, a successful procedure means the joint can bear weight better, is more stable, and is no longer painful. Risks associated with arthrodesis include pain at the site of the fusion, nerve injury, infection, and a failed fusion, which requires an additional surgery.

Osteotomy

Sometimes arthritis affects certain joints in a way that causes them to become misaligned, resulting in a deformity. A realignment, or osteotomy, of a joint can reverse a deformity. The knee is the joint most often realigned, and this allows the leg to remain vertical instead of leaning forward. Hip realignment can be beneficial if done early in the disease. An osteotomy can provide pain relief, but it is typically best performed in relatively young people whose knees still have good range of motion and are not completely overcome with osteoarthritis.

Resection

This procedure involves removing part or all of a bone. It used to be performed much more frequently to relieve pain and improve function in the hands and wrists in the early stages of rheumatoid arthritis. Today it is mostly done on the feet or along with joint replacement.

Spinal Surgery

Osteoarthritis can cause spinal stenosis or lateral canal stenosis, a condition in which the space for the spinal cord or the nerves emerging from it is compressed. If the stenosis is caused by bony spurs, a surgeon can do a procedure called decompression, in which he or she widens the space by removing tiny chips of bone. If the stenosis is caused by the protrusion of a disk, a surgeon may perform a diskectomy, which involves removing the part of the disk that is sticking out. In some patients, a disk affected by arthritis causes a significant amount of pain and fusing the two adjacent vertebrae can provide relief.

Synovectomy

This surgical procedure is usually performed in the wrist, elbow, or knee of people who have rheumatoid arthritis, and it may be done along with resection (see "Resection"). A synovectomy involves removing diseased synovium, the protective lining of a joint. When the damaged synovium is removed, it reduces inflammation, swelling, and pain. While a synovectomy may slow or prevent damage to the joint, the synovium can grow back after several years, and the problem may recur. Possible complications include a risk of bleeding into the joint and postoperative stiffness.

Washing Out

Sometimes bits of bone fragments collect in a joint, such as an elbow or knee, causing severe pain and limited movement. If this occurs, a surgeon may perform a washing-out procedure in which an arthroscope (a fiberoptic tube that has a camera at its tip) is threaded into the joint through a tiny incision. The physician then evaluates the joint area through the camera and uses instruments such as forceps to remove the bone fragments. He or she will also roughen the bone surface of the joint to help stimulate the formation of new cartilage. Washing out can reduce or eliminate pain, but it does not slow the arthritic process.

DID YOU KNOW?

There are several things you can do to get fit for surgery, including (1) get as much exercise as possible
(continued)

to improve your fitness and strength; (2) if you smoke, stop; (3) if you are overweight, lose weight; (4) avoid infections; and (5) tell your doctor and surgeon about any medications and supplements you are taking, as they could interfere with the surgery.

JOINT REPLACEMENT SURGERY

Joint replacement surgery, also known as arthroplasty, is the most common type of surgical procedure for arthritis. It is performed on hundreds of thousands of people every year in the United States. Total joint replacement is highly successful and can provide many years of stable, pain-free movement for patients who have osteoarthritis or rheumatoid arthritis.

Total joint replacement may involve the knee, hip, shoulder, wrist, ankle, elbow, and knuckles. Joint replacement surgery has continued to improve over the decades, and today it is highly successful, with minimal side effects and complications and rare breakage of the implants. The artificial joints are fixed into position either with or without cement, a fast-setting polymer that binds the implant to the bone and helps transmit the weight of the body between the two. Cementless joints usually have a porous surface that the surgeon fits next to the bone. Over time, the bone grows into the joint.

Generally, cementless joint replacements are believed to last longer than those that involve cement. Both types of replacements usually last at least 15 years, and some last longer. A downside of uncemented joint replacements is that patients usually require a longer recovery time. The question of "cement or no cement?" will be one you will need to discuss with your surgeon.

SPOTLIGHT ON RESEARCH

A yearlong trial using stem cell therapy for osteoarthritis is slated for launch at the end of 2010. Experts believe it could be the first step toward new treatments that would avoid the need for joint replacement surgery and painkilling drugs for people who have osteoarthritis. The new therapy involves mixing stem cells with young cartilage cells and then injecting them into the patients' joints. Seventy patients with knee osteoarthritis are planned to be enrolled into the study. The trial is part of a five-year research program.

Hip Replacement

The natural hip consists of a ball-and-socket joint. The head of the thigh bone (femur) moves in a socket in the pelvis. The joint is held together by muscles, tendons, and ligaments. In people with osteoarthritis, the hip joint can wear out and become stiff and painful, signaling the need for a replacement when function and/or pain becomes too great.

More than two hundred thousand Americans undergo total hip replacement surgery each year. In this procedure, the damaged or diseased head and neck of the femur are removed and replaced with artificial parts called the prosthesis. Damage and pain associated with osteoarthritis is the most common reason people chose hip replacement surgery, but rheumatoid arthritis, fracture, and bone tumors may also result in a breakdown of the hip joint and require surgical replacement.

Hip replacement surgery is recommended most often for people older than age 50, but individuals who have had rheumatoid arthritis from childhood or who developed it at an early age may need to undergo the procedure sooner. Total hip replacement has been extremely successful in allowing people to live active, independent, and more comfortable lives.

If you are contemplating hip replacement surgery with an orthopedic surgeon, there are a few factors to consider. One is the question of cement versus no cement. Because it takes a long time for natural bone to grow and attach to an artificial joint, you will need to limit your physical activities for up to three months if you choose an uncemented hip joint replacement. Another downside of an uncemented prosthesis is that it typically causes thigh pain during the first few months after surgery as the bone grows into the prosthesis.

Whether you choose cement or no cement, you will spend no more than three to five days in the hospital after your hip replacement and full recovery will take about three to six months, depending on the type of surgery, your overall health, and how your rehabilitation goes.

Another consideration is the type of hip replacement surgery your doctor will perform. Conventional surgery involves incisions based on the patient's size, as overweight and obese individuals typically require larger incisions. Minimally invasive surgery is a possibility for some patients, based on their health and weight. This type of surgery requires the use of less pain medication and results in a shorter postsurgery hospital stay, smaller surgical scars, and less blood loss during surgery. The possibility of minimally invasive surgery is something you should discuss with your surgeon.

According to the American Academy of Orthopaedic

Surgeons, about 90 percent of the more than 231,000 total hip replacements performed in the United States each year do not require revision. (A revision means a surgeon needs to replace the original artificial joint with a new one.) Revision surgery is becoming more common, especially because more people are choosing hip replacement surgery at a younger age. Because an artificial hip joint typically has a 15-to-20-year life, it is very possible that a 40-year-old individual will need revision surgery by the time he or she is 60 or 65.

While hip replacement surgery is usually successful, some problems can arise. The most common complication that may occur soon after surgery is hip dislocation. That's because the artificial ball and socket are smaller than the normal ones and the ball can become dislodged if the hip is in certain positions, such as pulling the knees up to the chest.

A later complication of hip replacement surgery is inflammation in the replacement area, which can eat away some of the bone and cause the implant to loosen. This can be treated with anti-inflammatory medications or revision surgery. Less common complications may include infection, blood clots, and excessive bone formation.

Of the hundreds of thousands of procedures performed each year, four to eight hundred people develop a fatal pulmonary embolism within the first three months after surgery. A pulmonary embolism is a blood clot that develops in a leg vein, breaks off, and travels to the lungs.

Some of these complications may require a patient to undergo revision surgery. Revision surgery is more difficult than first-time hip replacement surgery and the outcome is usually not as good, so you need to consider these facts when you are exploring your surgical options.

After undergoing hip replacement surgery, you will

need to talk to your doctor or physical therapist about an appropriate exercise program to help reduce stiffness and increase your flexibility and muscle strength. High-impact activities such as jogging, tennis, and racketball are generally discouraged, but walking, swimming, and stationary bicycling can be very beneficial.

Resurfacing a Hip Joint

Resurfacing a hip joint is an option for hip replacement in which the hip joint is relined rather than replaced. The orthopedic surgeon grinds down the surface of the affected ball in the hip and fits it with a metal cap. The cap fits into a metal shell that lines the hip socket and is supported by a stem in the neck of the femur.

Resurfacing a hip joint allows patients to keep their own hip joint as long as possible. Another advantage is that resurfacing results in metal-on-metal of a hard, biocompatible alloy that has very low rates of wear. A resurfaced hip, unlike a prosthetic hip joint, is also similar in size to the natural hip, which means there is less chance of dislocation.

Recovery time after hip joint resurfacing is less than for total hip replacement surgery, but you will still need some rehabilitation therapy. Most patients are able to return to everyday activities by three months postsurgery.

SPOTLIGHT ON RESEARCH

A study of nearly 3,100 patients who had undergone hip or knee replacement surgery found that

there may be a connection between the type of
anesthesia patients receive and the incidence of
surgical site infections. Of the 3,081 patients, 56
experienced a surgical site infection within 30 days
of their procedure. Of the 56 who had an infection,
33 had received general anesthesia, while the
remaining 23 patients had received epidural or
spinal anesthesia. Although this finding does not
prove general anesthesia causes more surgical site
infections, it is information patients who are
contemplating hip or knee replacement surgery
may want to consider when talking with their
surgeon about the use of anesthesia.

Knee Replacement

Knee replacement—total or partial—is one of the most
successful elective surgeries performed. The procedure
replaces severely damaged cartilage with a metal or plastic prosthesis that can function like a natural knee joint.
Nearly all of the three hundred thousand total knee replacement surgeries conducted in the United States each
year are done in the elderly, although the surgery can be
done in adults of any age. Because younger patients tend
to be more active than older ones, those men and women
may need to undergo a repeat surgery when their prosthesis wears out after 15 years or so.

About 90 percent of adults who have total knee replacement experience freedom from pain and improved function
and mobility for about 15 years after surgery. In some cases,
surgeons need to replace only part of the joint. This procedure is called a partial or unicompartmental knee replacement. The best candidate for partial knee replacement is an

individual who has arthritis in only one section (compartment) of the knee and who is not obese. Individuals who are younger than 60 and who have a sedentary lifestyle may also benefit from this procedure. About seventy-five hundred such procedures are done each year in the United States. A drawback of partial replacement is that future surgical procedures may be more difficult to perform.

If you are experiencing pain in both knees and X-rays show severe arthritis in both joints, your doctor may suggest replacing both knees at the same time. Called bilateral knee replacement, it reduces the amount of time you will spend in rehab. To qualify for bilateral knee replacement, you must be in good health and free of heart and lung disease, among other conditions.

If you are contemplating knee replacement surgery, one topic that should come up is whether you can undergo minimally invasive surgery. This approach allows the surgeon to use smaller incisions, which involve less invasion of your soft tissues. Minimally invasive surgery can be more difficult to perform, however, and only some patients are candidates. If you are bowlegged or you have had previous major surgery, for example, you may not qualify. Your orthopedic surgeon will determine whether you can undergo such a procedure. In some hospitals, computer-assisted surgery is available. This approach allows a much more precise alignment of the implant, which may improve the patient's long-term success.

The typical postsurgery hospital stay for total knee replacement is two to four days; and for bilateral knee replacement, four to six days. If you have a partial knee replacement, an overnight stay is usually all that's necessary. Physical therapy begins in the hospital and continues at a rehabilitation center and at home. You will need to use crutches or a walker for about three to six weeks after surgery.

A Knee Replacement Story

If you met Howard today, you would not know that two years ago he could barely climb the four steps on his front porch in Virginia. By age 53, Howard had tried nearly every drug and several nutritional and herbal supplements on the market to deal with his osteoarthritis in his knees and he had had some success with acupuncture and hydrotherapy for a while. "But it just wasn't enough," says the construction foreman who has run his own business for three decades. "I'm visiting job sites every day, climbing stairs, walking over rough terrain, and getting in and out of the truck. The pain and stiffness made it impossible for me to continue working. And I love my job. I didn't want to give it up."

Fortunately, Howard's health, except for the arthritis, was excellent, so he opted for bilateral knee replacement, even though he knew it meant he would be recovering for many months. "Better being off the job for a few months than forever," he said. Since he was a candidate for minimally invasive surgery, he chose that option, and after the surgery he attacked his rehabilitation with vigor. Two months after his surgery Howard was visiting his job sites from the comfort of his partner's truck, and six months postsurgery Howard was back on the job sites, able to comfortably do about half his presurgery routines.

"The doctor says if I'm smart and don't try to run any marathons, I'll be fully back on the job by one year," says Howard. "I feel like I got my life back after this surgery."

Other Joint Replacements

Has rheumatoid arthritis damaged your ankle? Ankle replacement surgery is becoming more common. The best candidate for ankle replacement is someone who is older than 50, who is not too heavy, and who is not extremely active. Although patients who undergo ankle replacement can regain much of the mobility in the ankle, it is not 100 percent. Activities that are not recommended after ankle replacement are those that involve repetitive pounding, such as running, or a job that includes heavy labor. Anyone who has poor circulation in the leg, diabetes, or a nerve condition is not a good candidate.

Replacement of the shoulder joint is performed for both osteoarthritis and rheumatoid arthritis. The shoulder joint is a ball-and-socket arrangement much like the hip, although the socket is not so deep. Around the shoulder the rotator cuff muscles stabilize the joint. A procedure called a half-joint replacement (hemiarthroplasty) is frequently done for people with rheumatoid arthritis when the rotator cuff muscles are not in good shape. A hemiarthroplasty is usually effective in relieving pain, although the surgery may not improve the shoulder's range of movement. Total shoulder replacement is usually performed when the joint is damaged in osteoarthritis. The success of the surgery usually depends on how much bone is still in the socket, as this is the factor that will determine how well the replacement can be secured.

Only a small number of orthopedic surgeons perform elbow replacement surgery. When it is done, it is performed for individuals who have rheumatoid arthritis in that joint and it can provide significant improvement in quality of life. Even less common is wrist replacement, and it is still considered somewhat experimental.

Replacement of knuckles is common in people who have rheumatoid arthritis. Surgeons sometimes replace these joints with silicone-like spacers that can provide significant relief from pain while also improving function of the hand. Individuals who have deforming and debilitating rheumatoid arthritis of the knuckles can benefit greatly from this procedure.

GOUT SURGERY

Most people who have gout can treat it successfully using medications and watching their diet. Some patients, however, have recurring attacks for 10 years or longer, and by that time the uric acid crystals have accumulated in the joints to form nodules called tophi. These nodules can cause infection, pain, deformed joints, and pressure, and if the medications your doctor prescribes cannot shrink or eliminate the tophi you may need surgery to remove them. Recovery from surgery varies. Most people are up and walking with crutches within two days, but you should plan to have limited mobility for about two weeks.

PREPARING FOR SURGERY

In most cases, surgical procedures for arthritis are elective surgery, so you have time to prepare. Some things you and your doctor will need to address are any potential health problems, such as high blood pressure, asthma, or diabetes, and how the surgery will affect these conditions. If you are overweight, losing weight can be very beneficial, especially if you are having a hip or knee replacement, as reduced weight can improve your recovery time and results.

To help you prepare for what you should know before and after surgery, here is a list of questions you can ask yourself and your surgeon.

Questions to Ask Before Surgery

- Do I understand the surgical procedure? Are there written materials, videos, or other information I can see?

- Do I need to stop taking any medications or supplements before I undergo the procedure?

- Can I speak with other patients who have had this procedure done?

- How long will I need to stay in the hospital after surgery?

- How much pain is normally associated with this procedure? How long will the pain last? How will the pain be treated?

- What risks are associated with the surgery?

- What risks are associated with my not having the surgery?

- Will I need to lose weight before I undergo the procedure?

- What are the chances that I will need additional surgery?

- What benefits can I expect from the surgery?

- What type of exercise will I be able to do after the surgery?

- How soon after the surgery will I begin rehabilitation therapy? How long will I need to do rehab? Can I do rehab at home?

- Will I need any special assistance at home after the surgery? Will I need any special equipment or devices to help me?

- How long will it take for me to return to my everyday activities, such as climbing stairs, driving, having sex, going back to work?

- How often will I need to make follow-up visits?

Answers to these questions—and perhaps others that may come to mind as you read through these—can help you feel confident going into the procedure and when you are recovering.

AFTER SURGERY

Congratulations! Undergoing a surgical procedure is a big step in improving your symptoms and enhancing your quality of life. The "real" work begins with your rehabilitation and recovery. Your rehab efforts will pay off if you are dedicated and patient. The amount of time you will need for rehab and recovery will vary, depending on the procedure you have had. Rehabilitation after knee replacement surgery, for example, requires more effort than rehab after hip replacement, and your recovery time will be longer as well. Rehabilitation of a surgically repaired joint can be tedious, but with the help of your physical or occupational therapist you can begin to enjoy the benefits of the surgery almost immediately, if only in small increments at first.

Only a small part of your rehab takes place in the hospital or your therapist's office, however. The real work is at home, where you will need to follow the exercise program designed for you. The benefits will be in proportion to the amount of work you do.

BOTTOM LINE

When other treatment options have not provided relief from symptoms of arthritis, surgery may be desirable. Fortunately, the available surgical procedures are largely effective and can provide the majority of patients with a better quality of life.

CHAPTER TEN

Food and Nutrition for Arthritis

What impact does the food you eat have on arthritis? Are there certain foods that trigger symptoms? How about foods that might make you feel better? These and other questions about the effect of diet on arthritis are often asked by people who have osteoarthritis, rheumatoid arthritis, and gout.

Experts generally agree that people who have arthritis need to follow the same type of well-balanced, nutritious diet that is good for everyone: lots of fresh fruits and vegetables, low-fat dairy, oily fish, whole grains and legumes, lean meat and poultry, and easy on fried foods, sugar, and refined foods. However, others insist that while this is good advice, people with arthritis may benefit by making some changes in their diet, changes that substitute or eliminate foods that may trigger inflammation and pain.

For now, there is limited scientific evidence that certain special diets—those that focus on several foods and/or eliminate many others, for example—can reduce symptoms of arthritis, although the anecdotal claims are plentiful. Rather than say such diets are not effective, however, let's say that everyone's body chemistry is different and that what works for one person may not work for another. Although special diets do not always offer much relief for people who have arthritis, the fact is that these diets frequently benefit some patients. A general rule is that if you choose a diet plan that involves eliminating some foods or adding others, as long as the end result is a menu that provides adequate nutrition and you do not have other health conditions that would be negatively impacted by the diet, then why not give it a go? You may be pleasantly surprised!

With these thoughts in mind, here are a few dietary approaches that may improve your symptoms and your quality of life. I suggest you keep a food diary to track any changes you make in your diet and your responses to them, because you may find a whole new way of eating that makes you feel better.

BASIC HEALTHY DIET FOR ARTHRITIS

Whether or not you decide to try a special diet for arthritis, you should still be familiar with the basic healthy eating plan that will ensure you get the right nutrients while maximizing your chances of fighting the symptoms of arthritis. Then, if you want to elaborate or make changes to that diet, you can do so along with the guidance of your healthcare provider.

Concentrate on Carbohydrates

Carbohydrates are your main source of energy and should make up the majority (55 to 60 percent) of your caloric intake, so you want them to come from the best sources. Those sources are foods that contain complex carbohydrates, such as whole grains, legumes, fruits, and vegetables, because they are digested slowly and give you a steady source of energy. Simple carbohydrates, including sugary foods and baked goods made with white flour, cause a sharp increase in energy, accompanied by a rise in blood sugar levels, followed by a "crash" and low energy.

Complex carbohydrates also contain fiber, which is important for digestion and intestinal health, which in turn impacts overall health. Fiber helps lower cholesterol levels and makes you feel full, which can help you eat less and lose excess pounds. Because being overweight places stress on arthritic joints, fiber can be your weight-loss friend!

Hold the Fat

Many health experts and organizations, including the American Heart Association, recommend that people limit fat intake to no more than 30 percent of their calories. No more than 10 percent should be saturated fat (e.g., meat, dairy products), and trans fat should be avoided as much as possible. If your daily caloric intake is 2,000 calories, 30 percent equals 600 calories from fat per day. If you break that down into grams of fat per day, it equals 67 grams (9 calories per gram of fat: 600 divided by 9 equals 67 grams).

All of this is not so hard to do if you choose low-fat meats and dairy products, reduce the amount of red meat and pork in your diet, and limit your use of added fats, oils, and salad dressings. Make it a habit to read nutritional labels on foods, as you may be surprised how much fat is in some foods. The amount of fat shown on nutritional labels is in grams, so once you know how many grams of fat you should limit yourself to each day, the rest is easy!

Eat a Variety of Foods

Variety is not only the spice of life; it is also good for your health. A healthful diet includes foods from all the food groups: fruits and vegetables; grains and cereals; beans and legumes, meat, and/or soy; and dairy. A variety is necessary to help ensure your body gets all the nutrients it needs.

When you are in pain, have limited mobility, or feel tired or depressed, it can be difficult to be motivated to prepare a variety of foods. Good nutrition is too important for you to neglect, so if you are having trouble getting a varied diet, talk to your health-care provider or a nutritionist. He or she may be able to help you directly, or you can contact your local chapter of the Arthritis Foundation and ask for guidelines on diet. (Also see "Resources.")

Limit Sugar, Salt, and Alcohol

Prepared and processed foods are great hiding places for excessive amounts of sugar and salt. Once again, it pays to read nutritional labels to uncover the amount of sugar and salt in the foods you choose. Too much sugar not only contributes to weight gain; it also provides empty calories when your body needs essential nutrients.

Excess salt (sodium) intake is also not healthy, as it can cause your body to retain fluids, which can increase how you perceive pain, and raise your blood pressure. Check out food labels for excess sodium and choose low-sodium foods or, better yet, select whole foods, which are free of added salt and naturally delicious!

SPOTLIGHT ON RESEARCH

Here is an interesting study, published in *Rheumatology* (July 2010), in which scientists discovered that drinking alcohol frequently may reduce the severity of symptoms of rheumatoid arthritis. The Sheffield University team found that individuals with the disease who drank alcohol on more than 10 days in the last month showed less joint damage, inflammation, pain, swelling, and disability than those who never drank alcohol. Why? One study author, Dr. James Maxwell, noted that "there is some evidence to show that alcohol suppresses the activity of the immune system, and that this may influence the pathways by which RA develops." Moderation, however, is still key.

FOOD ALLERGIES AND RHEUMATOID ARTHRITIS

Have you ever wondered why your joints feel more stiff, achy, or painful after you eat? If this has happened to you—or continues to occur—you may have also wondered if certain foods are contributing to these feelings. Scientists at the University of Oslo are among experts who believe that antibodies (proteins that attack and kill foreign substances) in the intestinal tract may cause inflammation in people who have rheumatoid arthritis. Although their work focused on testing patients' intestinal fluids in test tubes, these scientists did find that people who have rheumatoid arthritis have higher levels of antibodies to proteins from cow's milk, cereal, chicken eggs, cod, and pork than people without the disease.

This is a strong indication of a link between food intolerance/allergies and inflammation associated with rheumatoid arthritis. In an article in *Arthritis Today,* Jonathan Brostoff, DM, professor of allergy and environmental health at Kings College London, noted that "the gut is the first site of exposure to food, and the immune system in the gut is the first to recognize potential allergens." An allergic reaction to food occurs when the immune system incorrectly believes that something you ate is harmful. That's when your immune system steps in to protect you by producing immunoglobulin E (IgE antibodies) against the food. This sets off a chain reaction that causes symptoms. In some people the proteins and antibodies cling together and circulate throughout the body. If they get into the joints, they can contribute to inflammation.

Elimination Diet

The best way to determine whether certain foods cause inflammation for you is to try an elimination diet. Dr. Brostoff conducted a study in which he found that more than 33 percent of people with rheumatoid arthritis reported less morning stiffness and pain and experienced better range of motion felt better overall when they followed the standard Stone Age diet, which consists of fruit, vegetables, meat, and fish, for one month.

To conduct an elimination diet, you remove specific foods or ingredients from your diet that you believe may be causing or contributing to your arthritis symptoms. The Stone Age diet is a common approach, because it eliminates the common allergy-causing foods, including milk, eggs, nuts, wheat, and soy.

While on an elimination diet, you need to read food

labels carefully for suspected ingredients. You should also keep a food diary to record the foods you eat and any reactions you may have to any of them. If you stop eating a certain food and your symptoms decrease or go away while you are following this diet, it is likely that food is a cause of your problems.

To ensure you get a sufficient amount of nutrition while following an elimination diet, you should work with a knowledgeable professional, such as a nutritionist or dietician, who can help you plan your meals. After you have stayed on the elimination diet for two to four weeks, your doctor will ask you to gradually reintroduce the foods that you eliminated during your diet, one at a time. Record each food that you reintroduce and whether you experience any symptoms. Your doctor will likely ask you to eliminate that food item again to see if your symptoms disappear.

Sometimes there are emotional and physical factors that can affect the diet's results, so an elimination diet is not foolproof. For example, if you believe you are allergic to a certain food, your response could be a psychological one rather than a real allergic reaction. However, an elimination diet can also be very useful in discovering one or more foods that, once avoided, could significantly improve your life.

THE NIGHTSHADE DIET

One of the most popular and familiar diets associated with arthritis is the nightshade diet, in which vegetables that belong to the nightshade family—tomatoes, potatoes, eggplant, and some peppers—are avoided. Although these foods are a great source of nutrients, some people find that these foods trigger flares of pain and inflammation.

Felicia is one such individual. "I had a doctor tell me I was imagining that tomatoes and peppers were causing me to have more pain and swelling," she says. "And believe me, I love tomatoes, so it was not easy for me to stop eating them. But I tried eliminating nightshade vegetables and then adding them back into my diet, and the impact was clear. I think it's a small price to pay to feel better."

Experts are not certain why nightshade vegetables seem to trigger symptoms in some people. One hypothesis is that the vegetables contain substances that act as neurotoxins, which can trigger pain, inflammation, and swelling.

VEGAN DIET

One dietary approach that has proved beneficial, especially for people who have rheumatoid arthritis, is vegan. A vegan eating plan includes fruits, vegetables, grains, legumes, seeds, and cereals, while avoiding all animal products, including meat, poultry, fish, eggs, and dairy foods. While this approach may sound difficult on the surface, the wide availability of meat and dairy alternatives on the market today can make a vegan diet an easier transition for those who want to try it.

One 2002 study evaluated the effect of a very low-fat vegan diet on people who had moderate to severe rheumatoid arthritis. The participants followed the diet for four weeks, and all of them enjoyed a significant reduction in all their symptoms. In another study, patients who followed a gluten-free vegan diet also had improvement in signs and symptoms of rheumatoid arthritis. In a stricter study, patients with rheumatoid arthritis who followed a raw-food vegan diet experienced significant improvement in joint stiffness and pain.

One reason some experts believe a vegan diet can be

so beneficial for rheumatoid arthritis patients is that it is low in fat and it can also alter the composition of fats in the body, which in turn can impact the immune processes that influence arthritis. The omega-3 fatty acids in vegetables, as well as the near lack of saturated fat in the diet, are also factors that can benefit arthritis patients. People who switch to a vegan diet also frequently lose weight, which contributes to an improvement in symptoms as well. The high level of antioxidants associated with a vegan diet can help neutralize free radicals, those cell-damaging molecules that can attack the joints.

Neal Barnard, M.D., founder and president of the Physicians Committee for Responsible Medicine and author of *Foods That Fight Pain,* presents a program that arthritis patients can try. For four weeks, individuals can eat generous amounts of foods from the pain-safe list (see "Pain-Safe Foods") while also completely avoiding any foods that may trigger arthritis symptoms. Pain-free foods virtually never contribute to arthritis.

PAIN-SAFE FOODS

Brown rice
Dried and cooked fruits: cherries, cranberries, pears, prunes (avoid bananas, citrus, peaches, tomatoes)
Cooked green, yellow, and orange vegetables (artichokes, asparagus, broccoli, chard, collards, lettuce, spinach, string beans, summer or winter squash, sweet potatoes, tapioca, taro)

(continued)

Water, plain or carbonated
Condiments: modest amounts of salt, maple syrup,
   vanilla extract

After you have followed this diet for four weeks, if
your symptoms have improved or disappeared the next
step is to identify which one or more foods trigger your
symptoms. You can do this by reintroducing the foods
you stopped eating during the previous four weeks.

Dr. Barnard recommends avoiding meat, poultry, fish,
dairy products, and eggs completely and not reintroducing them back into your diet. These foods often are major
triggers of arthritis symptoms, and they also prompt hormone imbalances that can contribute to joint pain and
other health problems.

It is important to reintroduce each food one at a time,
every two days. If your symptoms flare up, eliminate the
food that seems to have caused the problem and allow
your joints to cool down. After your symptoms improve,
reintroduce another food. Wait at least two weeks before
you try a problem food a second time.

MAJOR ARTHRITIS TRIGGERS

Dairy products
Corn
Meats
Wheat, oats, rye
Eggs

Citrus fruits
Potatoes and tomatoes
Nuts
Coffee

GOUT DIET

A gout diet is typically one that significantly limits or
eliminates foods that contain purines. Uric acid is a waste
product that is left over from metabolism of purines, and
the accumulation of uric acid results in gout. Foods that
are especially rich in purines include liver, kidney, brain,
meat extracts, meats, and shellfish. To help prevent or
avoid repeat attacks of gout, it is also best to avoid or reduce your intake of beverages that contain fructose, and
alcohol consumption also should be minimized. The following foods may be eaten in moderation if you have gout:
asparagus, cauliflower, kidney and lima beans, mushrooms,
peas, spinach, whole-grain breads and cereals, and white
poultry meats.

ALKALINE DIET

The thesis of the alkaline diet is that both osteoarthritis
and rheumatoid arthritis are caused by the presence of
too much acid in the body and that the pH produced by
your diet should be similar to the pH level of your blood
(7.36). If you have an improper pH balance, it can lead to
various diseases, including arthritis. Therefore, the recommendations for those who wish to try this diet is to eat
75 to 80 percent alkaline foods and 20 to 25 percent acid
foods. Common alkaline foods include vegetables, nuts,

grains, and certain fruits (e.g., lemons, limes, grapefruit). Foods that form acid include refined and processed foods, dairy, sugar, meat, caffeine, alcohol, and saturated fats. Although there are no scientific studies to support the use of this diet for arthritis, some people say they feel better when they tip the scale in favor of alkaline foods.

OMEGA-3 FATTY ACIDS

A diet that contains foods rich in omega-3 fatty acids can benefit those who have arthritis, and here's why. (Note: I discuss omega-3 fatty acid supplements in chapter 7, but here I want to discuss their role in diet.) Omega-3 fatty acids are considered essential, which means they are necessary for human health, but because the body can't manufacture them, you must get them (preferably) through food or in supplements. Rich sources of omega-3s include fish such as salmon, tuna, herring, sardines, and halibut and other foods from the sea, including algae and krill. Foods that are considered a good or very good source include flaxseed and flaxseed oil, walnuts, and soybeans. If you want to benefit from this essential fatty acid, include at least one serving of an omega-3 food each day, including at least two servings of fish each week.

Many studies have examined the impact of essential fatty acids, especially omega-3 fatty acids, on both osteoarthritis and rheumatoid arthritis. One study, for example, found that the omega-3 fatty acid eicosapentaenoic acid (EPA) was more effective than the other two main omega-3s—docosahexaenoic acid (DHA) and alpha-linolenic acid. Omega-3 fatty acids inhibit the action of substances that cause inflammation, including prostaglandins and leukotrienes. Including omega-3 foods in your diet can also help reduce the number of tender joints and morning stiffness and allow you to reduce or even eliminate your use of arthritis medications.

BOTTOM LINE

Making modifications to your diet could very well provide you with relief from arthritis symptoms. Although there are not a great number of scientific studies to support dietary changes for arthritis patients, the ones that exist are largely positive, while the number of anecdotal reports are impressive. As Pauline, a 43-year-old woman with rheumatoid arthritis, reported in her support group, "My doctors told me changing my diet probably wouldn't do much to help my arthritis. They were right: it helped a *lot*. Once I stopped eating dairy products and added fish and flaxseed to my diet, my symptoms improved significantly. So my suggestion is, try making dietary changes. What do you have to lose? Probably some nasty symptoms, that's what!"

CHAPTER ELEVEN

Daily Living with Arthritis

When you have arthritis, the phrase "hopping out of bed in the morning" has its own special meaning. The pain, limited mobility, joint stiffness (especially in the morning), inflamed joints, and other symptoms of arthritis can take their toll even before you get out of bed each day. Thus those symptoms most certainly have an impact on the way you go about your daily life, whether that means taking care of your children, going out to work, running errands, socializing, or any combination of these and other activities.

Although the challenges associated with living with arthritis can be daunting, they also can be managed, even conquered, if you seek out and take advantage of resources from the community, family, and friends and from within yourself. In this chapter I discuss how to make things easier, safer, and more pleasurable in many different areas of your life by offering tips, guidelines, and resources you may not have realized are at your disposal.

ASSISTIVE DEVICES

Do you have trouble opening jars, bending over to pick up objects, or keeping your balance in the bathroom? When you have arthritis, often seemingly simple movements and tasks can become difficult, even impossible, to perform safely or with confidence. Assistive devices not only make a variety of tasks easier; they also help preserve your joints, extend your range of motion, reduce pain, and help eliminate the chance for injury.

There are assistive devices for tasks you need to perform at home and at work and for leisure. Here are just a few you can consider. Information on finding these and other devices is in the "Resources" section at the end of this book.

- **Bathroom.** Safety is an important issue in the bathroom. You may want to install tub and shower bars and handrails that will provide you with stability when getting in and out of the tub or shower. A grab bar next to the toilet may also be helpful, as well as a raised toilet seat, which can make it easier to get up from the toilet. Some faucet handles or levers can be a challenge to use if your hands are affected by arthritis. It may be necessary to change the faucets to a type that does not require you to grip and turn them. While you are in the tub or shower, using a shower chair can make you feel much more secure and the experience a much safer one.

- **Bedroom.** Arthritic fingers can have difficulty doing buttons and using zippers, and putting on shoes can be an Olympic event. Look for zipper pulls and buttoning aids that can help you with dressing challenges. An option to buttons, snaps, and zippers is Velcro fasteners. You can customize your favorite clothing with Velcro. A long-handled shoehorn can make it much easier to put on shoes.

If getting in and out of bed is a problem, a rail can be fitted to the frame.

- **Kitchen.** Items that can assist with food preparation are especially important, because frustration with making and cooking food often means some people do not get the proper nutrition because cooking is too much trouble. Dozens of special devices are available to help in the kitchen, including grips that make it easier to open jars and take stress off the fingers and built-up handles to make utensils easier to grasp. You may also want to turn to items such as lightweight cooking pots or a Crock-Pot, wide-handled peelers, knives with upright handles, easy-grip cups and glasses, scoop plates and bowls, and teapot tippers. An item called a reach extender—a rod with a trigger-controlled grasp at the far end—allows you to reach up to 30 inches and pick up small objects, such as a box of cereal out of a cupboard. A reach extender is a very handy item that can be used anywhere in the house, but it is limited to picking up light items.

- **On the job.** You may benefit from some adjustments or changes to your work space, such as adjustable chairs and work surfaces and hands-free headsets. An occupational therapist can work with you to decide what type of modifications can help you. (See "Returning to Work" later in this chapter.)

- **Outside/leisure.** There's no reason to give up hobbies and leisure activities that you have always enjoyed. If you like to work in the garden, for example, and bending over is now a problem, you can use a kneeler or a lightweight portable seat or walker with a seat on it. If holding a book is painful, you can get a book holder that can be used while sitting or reading in bed. If card games are a favorite, there are card holders and shufflers. Grip bars can be installed in a car to make getting in and out easier.

Splints, Braces, and Walking Support

Sometimes you may need something that physically supports and protects your joints. That's when your physical therapist or doctor may recommend a splint or brace. These support devices can be used on the wrist, hands, fingers, knees, and ankles and, depending on where the splint is, can help you walk, grip, handle objects, and ease pain and swelling. Splints can be custom made or purchased from a pharmacy or medical supply store. If you choose to buy your own splint, be sure to consult a healthcare professional first so you purchase the right item.

To be most effective, the splint or brace should not only cover the arthritic joint but extend past the joint as well. This helps to limit joint motion and protects the joint. A knee brace, for example, stabilizes the joint and gives more structure to it. If your knee tends to go to the side, the brace would prevent this, thus reducing friction and decreasing pain.

If you have painful knee and hip joints, a cane or walker could be a great help, in not only reducing the stress on these joints but also providing you with security against losing your balance and suffering a fall and possible fracture. All canes and walkers are not alike, so be sure to consult your physical therapist or doctor when choosing walking support.

Resources for assistive devices can be found in the "Resources" section at the back of the book.

SPOTLIGHT ON RESEARCH

A recent study (April 2010) showed that use of an ordinary heel lift or other corrective device for a shoe can help prevent or relieve knee osteoarthritis. Why? Because it can correct a leg length discrepancy, a condition that affects about 50 percent of Americans. Yet leg length discrepancy is something few people have ever had diagnosed or corrected. Not everyone who has this condition will suffer with knee osteoarthritis, but even a slight imbalance can place undue stress and strain on your joints. Therefore, it can be well worth having your doctor check for a possible leg length discrepancy.

HOW TO PROTECT YOUR JOINTS

Protecting your joints against stress, strain, and injury is essential, as it can prolong your ability to function, minimize pain, and allow you to live your life more fully. Joint protection is all about learning new ways to use your joints in more healthful ways. It can take some time to incorporate these changes into your life, but as you do, you will likely see how they will begin to come naturally, because they will feel better than doing things the "old" way.

- Avoid straining your neck by placing items you need to read or work on at eye level. Looking up and down for long periods of time places excessive stress on the neck.

- Put your larger joints to work rather than your smaller, weaker ones. For example, if you have arthritis in your fingers, carry shopping bags using your forearms or palms. Hint: Use canvas shopping bags that have wide straps or handles. Plastic bags from groceries and other stores can dig into your hands and arms, and they are not sturdy or safe.

- Use two hands instead of one, such as when holding a glass or cup or lifting a pan from the stove.

- Use long-handled reaching devices and tools when doing housework, gardening, and retrieving objects.

- Wear thick gloves or use a thick kitchen glove when you need to lift or move a heavy pot, hold a tool, or grip another type of object.

- Bend at the knees and straighten your legs while keeping your back straight if you need to lift objects. Also make a note when you do need to lift things: is there some way you can rearrange (or better yet, have someone else rearrange for you) items in your home so you don't need to bend or lift them? In the kitchen, for example: rearrange items you use often, such as pots or dishes, at a level that limits stress and strain on your joints.

- Rise from a seated position by sliding forward to the chair's edge while keeping your feet flat on the floor. Use your palms to push against the chair's seat or arms.

- Have your leg length checked. About 50 percent of people have a discrepancy in leg length, and although it can be very small, it can be enough to place additional and unnecessary stress on your joints, especially your knees. A recent study showed that correcting leg length discrepancy can both prevent and effectively treat knee osteoarthritis.

- Do not kneel or squat, because these positions place excessive strain on the knees and hips. If you want to do something that requires kneeling or squatting, such as gardening, use a portable seat or a walker with a seat.

- Maintain good posture. This avoids putting stress on your joints. Movement therapies such as the Alexander Technique and Feldenkrais Method can help with posture (see chapter 5).

- Use a cane or walker if necessary to reduce stress on your knees and hips when walking.

- Wear well-cushioned athletic shoes with good arch support and adequate space in the toe box (front of the shoe). In other words, high heels and shoes that are narrow in the toe area are not recommended. For women who want to wear dress shoes, heels should be no higher than one inch.

- Use wheels to move things. For example, you can use a cart with wheels to move laundry or other objects around the house. When going out, use a briefcase or suitcase with wheels to transport your laptop and office papers. Use a shopping cart in the store, even if you are getting only a few items.

SEX AND ARTHRITIS

When you are experiencing pain, discomfort, inflammation, and fatigue, it can be difficult to feel sexual. At the same time, you may want to engage in sexual relations with your partner, but your experience has been that it is uncomfortable or even painful, so you hold back. Your partner may or may not know how you feel, and therefore the most important thing to do is to communicate your feelings and concerns with your partner.

Arthritis can have a negative impact on your sexuality and how you feel about yourself as a sexual being, so it is important to address these issues with your partner. Some couples seek professional help from a therapist, marital counselor, or sex therapist, but many are able to work things out themselves. Often all that is needed is honest communication between partners about what they want, changes that they can make in how they are intimate that please both of them, and then trying different positions and ways to express their sexuality with each other.

Here are some tips you might try:

- Make a date. In fact, make dates on a regular basis. These dates will be times you and your partner set aside just for yourselves in a comfortable setting. Perhaps a quiet dinner, a picnic, a walk in the park. Make the times special for just the two of you, a time you can communicate without pressure.

• If you are taking medication for arthritis, take it at a reasonable time before sexual activity so you can be as pain free as possible.

• Explore new positions for sexual intercourse and/or new ways to please each other when intercourse is not possible.

• Take care of yourself. Get a manicure; get a massage; pamper yourself. When you feel good about yourself, you alleviate stress, depression, and tension, which contribute to pain.

• Talk to a health professional or sexual counselor that both you and your partner feel comfortable with to help you with any issues you may be unable to resolve.

ARTHRITIS ON THE JOB

For many people who have been diagnosed with arthritis, continuing to work or starting a new job does not introduce any significant problems. Especially in the early stages of osteoarthritis or rheumatoid arthritis, most people can manage their symptoms well enough to work if they want or need to.

Sometimes, however, arthritis symptoms may make it difficult or impossible to perform some aspects of your job. If this is a concern, the first thing you need to know is that you have rights. According to the Americans with

Disabilities Act (ADA) of 1990, employers must make reasonable accommodations for employees in their current position or consider them for suitable vacancies within the company. You should become familiar with your rights under the Occupational Safety and Health Act (1970) and the ADA Accessibility Guidelines for Buildings and Facilities (1991, 2002). See "Resources" at the end of the book for information on where to access this information.

Oftentimes an employer and the employee work out an arrangement by making modifications to the employee's work site and hours. Depending on the type of work you do, here are some changes that could be considered:

- Assistive devices or equipment, such as a headset if holding a phone is difficult or an ergonomic chair, being made available by the employer

- Possible elimination from your job description of things that are no longer feasible for you to do and addition of other responsibilities

- A work schedule modification, such as working at home some or all days, going on a part-time basis, having more flexible hours, or changing to a different shift

- A switch to another position within the same organization

Returning to Work

If you have to take a significant amount of time off from work for, say, surgery or rehabilitation, talk to your doctor, surgeon, or other health professional who will be involved in your treatment about the amount of time you will need to be away from your job and any changes and limitations you can expect. You will then have reliable information to share with your employer so together you can make arrangements for your return to work. Your return to work may require some of the modifications discussed earlier. However, it is important that these issues be discussed before your planned absence from work so you will know where you stand and feel more secure about your future with your employer.

Brent, a 55-year-old administrator for an environmental consulting firm, had been suffering for several years with knee pain due to arthritis. When his doctor finally recommended knee replacement surgery, Brent was concerned about his job. "I like my job, and I need to work, so those are two very good reasons why I was a bit anxious about telling my boss I needed time off for the surgery and then wanted to come back, but I wasn't sure I could do full-time for a while."

Brent first spoke with his surgeon and gathered information about the surgery, rehabilitation, and recovery time. He then went to speak with his supervisor about his situation. "We worked out a great plan," says Brent. "I would be allowed to work at home during my recovery. All I needed was a computer and my cell phone. We agreed I'd do videoconferencing until I could return to the office."

DEPRESSION AND ARTHRITIS

If you experience chronic pain associated with rheumatoid arthritis, chances are you may also be experiencing symptoms of depression. Research shows that people who have rheumatoid arthritis are twice as likely to have depression as people who do not have the arthritic condition, yet they are also unlikely to tell their doctor about it.

In fact, a study published in *Arthritis Care and Research* reported that nearly 11 percent of patients who had rheumatoid arthritis had moderately severe to severe symptoms of depression and that only 20 percent of patients discussed their depression with their rheumatologists. Even when depression was brought up, it usually was not discussed at length.

Depression is not a problem just for people who have rheumatoid arthritis, however. Although depression is not usually associated with osteoarthritis, this form of arthritis can cause physical limitations that disrupt people's lives and affect their ability to remain independent or mobile, which can lead to depression.

If you are experiencing symptoms of depression (see "Symptoms of Depression"), talk to your rheumatologist or your primary care physician. Depression can cause you to not take proper care of yourself—to miss or stop taking your medication, lose sleep, and/or follow a poor diet, all of which will have a negative impact on your arthritis and overall health. Once you talk to your doctor, he or she can prescribe an appropriate antidepressant, and/or you may want to talk to a therapist or try herbal remedies (e.g., St. John's wort, SAM-e; see chapter 7). The first step, however, is to acknowledge that you are experiencing symptoms of depression and then seek help. Proper treatment of your depression can improve your arthritis and your quality of life.

SYMPTOMS OF DEPRESSION

The National Institute of Mental Health describes the following symptoms of depression:

• Difficulty making decisions, concentrating, remembering details

• Decline in energy; fatigue

• Feelings of hopelessness and/or pessimism

• Feelings of worthlessness, helplessness, and/or guilt

• Insomnia

• Restlessness, irritability

• Persistent anxiety, sadness, or feeling "empty"

• Loss of appetite or overeating

• Loss of interest in activities that were once pleasurable, including sex

• Persistent pain and/or digestive problems that do not improve even with treatment

• Thoughts of suicide, suicide attempts

HOW TO COPE WITH FATIGUE

While fatigue is not typically a symptom of osteoarthritis, it is common among people who suffer with rheumatoid arthritis. In fact, when inflammation is especially active, as during a flare-up, fatigue can be overwhelming. If you have ever experienced this fatigue, then you probably know that it can make it difficult to concentrate, make you less able to deal with pain, and send your emotions into a tailspin.

Inflammation is not the only cause of fatigue in arthritis patients. However, when fatigue does creep into your life, it is a sign that something is wrong, and that means you can take steps to do something about it. If you let fatigue take over your life, it can feed a cycle of depression, poor eating habits, sleep problems, an inability or unwillingness to exercise, and more fatigue. But you don't have to let fatigue take control of your life!

Your first step is to identify why you feel fatigue, and then you can take action. Here are some possible reasons for fatigue and actions you can take:

- **Flare-up of inflammation.** Possible solutions: increase your medication or try a different anti-inflammatory, such as omega-3 fatty acids.

- **Pushing yourself too hard.** Possible solutions: reduce the number of tasks or activities you try to do each day; get some temporary help with your tasks; take more breaks; make lists so you can stay on task.

- **Side effect of new medication.** Possible solution: check with your health-care provider if you have started a new medication, as fatigue may be a side effect. You may need to switch to another medication, reduce your dose, or even try a natural alternative.

- **Feeling depressed, stressed, and/or anxious.** Possible solutions: As these emotional challenges can easily drain your energy, try keeping a fatigue journal (see "A Fatigue Journal") to help identify the reasons for your feelings and sharing your concerns with your partner, a good friend or family member, or a therapist. Relaxation techniques such as yoga, meditation, and hypnotherapy may also help.

- **Poor sleep/insomnia.** Possible solutions: Ask your health-care provider to suggest a medication or natural sleep aid. You may also want to try some of the "Suggestions for a Good Night's Sleep."

- **Too little activity.** Possible solutions: Yes, because not getting enough exercise can cause fatigue, talk to your health-care provider or a physical therapist about establishing an exercise program for you. Ask a friend to join you if you need motivation.

A Fatigue Journal

Keeping a fatigue journal can help you identify the reasons why you experience fatigue. Some people find that while they are recording information about when they feel fatigue and what seems to trigger each episode, they learn other things about the disease that help them.

Carolyn, for example, decided to keep a fatigue journal after a friend, who like Carolyn also had rheumatoid arthritis, said it had helped her realize she was trying to do too much. "It became obvious when I saw it written down in black and white," she explained. "Once I accepted the fact that I did not need to be 'wonder mom' and that it actually was doing more harm than good, I began to prioritize my time, and I began to feel better."

Carolyn came to a different realization when she kept her journal: she saw that when she ate certain foods, especially those containing gluten, she felt much more tired and achy than when she avoided them. This discovery prompted her to talk to a nutritionist, who worked with her on an elimination diet (see chapter 10). "I found that along with certain foods bothering me, I had been worrying excessively about my condition," she said. "Like my friend Janet, when I was able to read what I had been doing I saw everything clearly. So keeping a journal really does work!"

SUGGESTIONS FOR A GOOD NIGHT'S SLEEP

- Establish a regular sleep routine: go to bed the same time each night and get up the same time each morning.

- Make sure your sleeping environment is comfortable and conducive to sleep. That means, make sure you have a comfy pillow and bedcoverings, there is no light in the room, the room is a satisfactory temperature, there are no distracting noises (some people, however, like white noise or soft music in the background).

(continued)

- Don't look at the clock. In fact, if there is a clock in your bedroom, turn it so you can't see it. If you wake up during the night or you can't sleep, "watching the clock" is stressful.

- If you smoke, quit, or at least do not smoke several hours before going to bed.

- Limit your use of alcohol, especially within two to three hours of going to bed. It may help you fall asleep, but when it begins to metabolize and you wake up you will likely have difficulty going back to sleep.

- Reduce or eliminate use of caffeinated beverages.

- Exercise every day, but not within two hours of going to bed. You may benefit, however, from gentle stretching before retiring, as it may help you to relax.

- Avoid eating a large meal two to three hours before retiring. If you feel hungry before bedtime, a light, low-fat snack or a cup of herbal tea (chamomile, valerian) may be helpful.

- Treat your pain if it is preventing you from falling asleep or staying asleep.

- Use prescribed sleep medications only as directed.

HOW TO HANDLE HOUSEHOLD TASKS

Cleaning, cooking, doing the laundry, ironing, running errands, picking up after your kids—routine household tasks can be a significant challenge when you have arthritis. All of these activities involve movements that can put a great deal of stress and strain on your joints, causing pain and stiffness, and draining you of your energy.

If you have a partner, children, or other family or friends who can help with some of your household tasks, by all means welcome their assistance! In fact, asking your children to help with household chores is an excellent way for them to learn responsibility and also appreciate that arthritis is a condition that can offer some challenges but ones that can be overcome.

Even if you do have help—and not everyone does—here are some things you can do to make household tasks and errands easier on your body:

- **Vacuuming.** When cleaning, remain in an upright position. A lightweight upright vacuum cleaner is easier and less stressful to use than a canister type. Make sure the model you get is not difficult to drag around and that you can manipulate any hand controls and change the bags without a problem. If your house has more than one floor, you may want to have a vacuum on each floor or have someone carry the vacuum upstairs for you.

- **Mopping and sweeping.** Again, keep in an upright posture and avoid strain on your back and other joints. If sweeping, use a long-handled dustpan to pick up the debris. Choose a mop that does not require use of a bucket. Consider using a steam cleaner instead of a mop.

- **Laundry.** If possible, use washing machines and dryers that load from the front, as they are easier to handle than top loaders. You may use a portable seat or chair so you can sit while loading and unloading the machines. Get a laundry cart on wheels so you don't need to carry the laundry around the house. If you have laundry to bring down steps, put it inside a pillowcase and toss it down the stairs.

- **Cooking.** Take advantage of the many kitchen tools specially made for people with arthritis, such as chunky-grip knives, peelers, and spoons. Use lightweight cooking pots and pans, preferably those that have two handles. Even if a pot has only one handle, use both hands when lifting and moving it. Make sure the handles of pots and pans have chunky-grip or other easy-grip covers, or use thick kitchen gloves for grasping items. To avoid having to pick up heavy pans of water, steam or microwave vegetables. You can use a steam basket that fits inside a saucepan and just remove the basket when the food is done, leaving the heavier pan to cool. Sit rather than stand when preparing food in the kitchen. If you need to move food, containers, or pots around the kitchen or into another room, use a wheeled cart.

- **Shopping.** If you have difficulty reaching items on the shelves and/or putting items into your cart and retrieving them, take someone with you when shopping or take advantage of Internet or home-delivery services. Many grocery stores allow you to fill out your shopping list online and then you have your food delivered to your home for a small charge. It is now possible to shop for just about anything online, from shampoo to lawn furniture to toasters. Whenever you do go out to shop, take advantage of disability parking privileges (handicapped parking permits) if you qualify. (Check with your health-care provider for certification and your state motor vehicle division for regulations.)

Overall, three general tips for handling household and other tasks are Prioritize, Plan, and Pace. If you are preparing a meal, for example, plan ahead and gather together all the ingredients and utensils you will need in one place so you have easy access. If you need to run several errands, plan your route so you expend the least amount of energy. At the same time, pace yourself. If you have six errands to run in one week, do not do them all in the same day. Prioritize them, then plan to complete them in two trips rather than one.

Beverly, a 45-year-old mother of three, says she found that posting a "Chore Calendar" on the refrigerator for her kids helped her feel less stressed about getting tasks done around the house. "I'm fortunate that my kids, ages nine, twelve, and thirteen, are old enough to understand that I have lots of rough days, and they are fairly good about pitching in. They know that if they need certain clothes laundered, they have to do it themselves. They load the dishwasher and empty it. If I'm too tired or hurting too much, I just close the kids' bedroom doors if the rooms are too messy. Messy rooms are not a big priority for me, and I've learned to let it go. They know I can't always run an errand for them, and they find ways to get around it. We've actually grown closer since I was diagnosed with rheumatoid arthritis. A blessing in disguise, I guess."

PREGNANCY AND ARTHRITIS

"I'm pregnant and I have arthritis. How will pregnancy affect my disease, and vice versa?" "I want to have a baby, but I have rheumatoid arthritis. Is it safe for me and my baby if I get pregnant?"

These and other questions about arthritis and pregnancy are important for women who have arthritis. Some women who have arthritis have even been advised to avoid pregnancy, because there is some uncertainly about how a rheumatic condition will affect the pregnancy and how pregnancy will impact the arthritis.

Impact of Rheumatoid Arthritis on Pregnancy

Is it more difficult to get pregnant if you have rheumatoid arthritis? Experts are uncertain whether the disease reduces fertility in women and men. Although women with rheumatoid arthritis do take longer to conceive than women without the disease, other factors such as inconsistent ovulation and a decreased sex drive may be explanations. Men who have rheumatoid arthritis can experience a temporary reduction in sperm count and function, decreased sex drive, and erection problems when they have flares of the disease.

Having rheumatoid arthritis does not seem to harm a developing fetus, even if a woman is experiencing active disease during pregnancy. The vast majority of pregnant women who have rheumatoid arthritis have a normal pregnancy without complications, although there is a slight risk of miscarriage and low–birth weight births.

The major concern associated with rheumatoid arthritis and pregnancy is the use of medications, including methotrexate and leflunomide, which can cause birth defects. These same medications may cause birth defects

even if they are taken by men who father children. Therefore, it is important for both women and men to talk to
their doctor if either partner is taking these or other drugs
for rheumatoid arthritis before pregnancy occurs.

Guidelines and Discussion

The College of Rheumatology offers some information
and guidelines for women with arthritis who are or who
want to become pregnant. You can review them and discuss your questions and concerns with your partner and
health-care providers so you can arrive at a decision that
is best for you.

- Any women who has arthritis and who is pregnant
  should be under the care of both an obstetrician
  and a rheumatologist, and these professionals need
  to maintain good communications with both the
  patient and each other, throughout the pregnancy
  and after.

- The impact of pregnancy on rheumatoid arthritis
  (and other rheumatic diseases) varies according
  to the condition. Between 70 and 80 percent of
  women with rheumatoid arthritis experience an
  improvement in their symptoms during pregnancy,
  and this allows many women to significantly reduce or even stop their arthritis medications while
  they are pregnant. Soon after delivery, however,
  symptoms tend to flare up. In the remaining 20 to
  30 percent, symptoms do not change or get worse.

- Six months prior to pregnancy, women who have
  rheumatic disease that is inactive or in remission
  and who have normal blood pressure and kidney

function are likely to have a successful pregnancy. However, women who have abnormal kidney function, uncontrolled blood pressure, or active rheumatic disease are often advised to avoid pregnancy.

• Women who want to become pregnant should have their rheumatoid arthritis under control for at least three to six months before getting pregnant. During that time, women should be counseled by a rheumatologist and an obstetrician, both of whom can help develop a plan to manage the disease and the pregnancy.

• Women who are at low risk of complications during pregnancy should still see their rheumatologist at three-month intervals during pregnancy.

• Women at high risk for complications should have an obstetric team that is familiar with high-risk pregnancies. Factors that make a pregnancy high risk include active rheumatoid arthritis, kidney impairment, heart conditions, pulmonary hypertension, restrictive lung disease, in vitro fertilization, multiple births, and a history of obstetric problems.

• It is best for women to avoid taking any medications until they have delivered their baby and have completed nursing. For women who need medication to keep their symptoms under control, the risk of uncontrolled disease must be weighed against potential risks to the unborn child. The list of drugs that obstetricians, internists, and rheumatologists generally agree are acceptable and not acceptable for women to use during pregnancy and lactation is provided here. If you are taking leflunomide, you need to stop taking this drug about two years before trying to conceive, because the medication has a very long half-life. You can talk to your health-care provider about ways to possibly "wash" the drug out of your system faster.

ACCEPTABLE ARTHRITIS DRUGS DURING PREGNANCY AND LACTATION

- Nonsteroidal anti-inflammatory drugs (NSAIDs) until week 32

- Sulfasalazine (Azulfidine)

- Hydroxychloroquine (Plaquenil)

- Corticosteroids (less than 10 milligrams daily when possible)

ARTHRITIS DRUGS ACCEPTABLE DURING PREGNANCY BUT NOT DURING LACTATION

- Azathioprine (Imuran®)

- Cyclosporine A

ARTHRITIS DRUGS UNACCEPTABLE DURING PREGNANCY AND LACTATION

- Methotrexate

- Cycophenolate (CellCept)

- Cyclophosphamide (Cytoxan®)

- Anti-TNF drugs (Enbrel®, HUMIRA®, REMI-CADE®)

- Rituximab (Rituxan®)

- Leflunomide (Arava®)

HOW TO FIND HELP AND SUPPORT

When you have arthritis, there are numerous sources of support, so you don't have to face your challenges alone. First, of course, you need to acknowledge your limitations and be willing to accept assistance without feeling guilty. Everyone needs a little help sometime!

Family and Friends

The first place many people turn to for help is family and friends. You may be surprised how willing people are to help if you just ask! Often other people do not realize you even need some assistance. You may feel more comfortable asking for help if you are prepared: decide exactly what you need to have done (e.g., grocery shopping on specific days, moving furniture, bringing your dog to the vet, changing lightbulbs that you can't reach) so the task is clearly defined. That way other people will know exactly what is needed and they can decide whether they can do it for you.

You!

Another person you can turn to for help is yourself. Yes, it is helpful if you learn as much as you can about your type of arthritis and all the ways you can manage it. Knowledge is power: although you may like and trust your doctor, that does not mean you cannot do some research on your own and learn about other alternative treatments and where you can access practitioners of those therapies. If your doctor is not comfortable helping you with pursuing other treatment options, then you may want to learn what you can and find health-care providers who will help you.

Support Groups

Research shows that arthritis support groups can boost mood, help people learn new coping skills, and help relieve pain. "My arthritis support group has been a lifesaver," says Georgia, a 48-year-old interior designer who was diagnosed with rheumatoid arthritis two years ago. "The companionship, great ideas, support, understanding—these are things I just don't get from other people as much as I do from the people in the group."

Many people who participate in arthritis support groups have a similar experience, but not everyone agrees. One criticism of support groups in general is that they can be a "pity party," attended by some people who complain but never seem to move forward. Rather than feel empowered, they dwell in their disease.

One benefit of support groups, however, is that in many cities and towns people have more than one group from which to choose. That means you will likely be able to visit the different gatherings in your area and find one that suits you. Some groups, for example, are moderated by professionals who have a structured format, while others are more informal and are peer or self-help, "run" by the participants.

When looking for an arthritis support group in your area, you can contact your local Arthritis Foundation chapter, ask your health-care provider, and contact local hospitals, which often host such meetings. Churches, community centers, and even people's homes are other locations where support group meetings can take place. The different types of support groups include:

- **Educational.** These groups feature an expert's presentation, often with question-and-answer sessions.

- **Closed.** Such groups are not open to the public unless you preregister. Closed groups require that you commit to attend a predetermined number of sessions.

- **Group therapy.** These groups are headed by a mental health professional and have specific therapeutic goals established and a certain time frame within which they expect to meet these goals. Group therapy sessions sometimes teach coping skills and relaxation techniques.

- **Peer.** These support groups are informal and led by fellow patients. Participants share their experiences and thus learn from one another.

Online Support Groups

Arthritis support groups found on Internet chat and forum sites are considered peer groups. Participating in these groups may help you feel connected with similarly minded folks 24 hours a day, seven days a week. Often online support groups for arthritis and related conditions also provide resource materials, videos, reading lists, the latest research information, and other items of interest. I have listed some online arthritis support groups and forums in the "Resources" section.

RESOURCES

Aids for Arthritis Inc.

35 Wakefield Drive
Medford NJ 08055
800-654-0707

http://www.aidsforarthritis.com/catalog/index.html

Offers many arthritis assistive devices for home and personal use

Comfort House

189-V Frelinghuysen Avenue
Newark NJ 07114
800-359-7701

http://www.comforthouse.com/dres.html

Assistive devices for home, outdoor (e.g., gardening), and personal use

ESI Ergonomic Solutions

4030 E. Quenton Drive, Suite 101
Mesa AZ 85215
800-833-3746

http://www.esiergo.com/

Provides products that add comfort, flexibility, and mobility to computer workstations

Life Solutions Plus

67 Wyndmere Way
Willow Street, PA 17584
877-785-8326

http://www.lifesolutionsplus.com

Good selection of arthritis assistive devices for home and personal use

EDUCATION AND SUPPORT GROUP INFORMATION

AcupressureOnline.org

http://www.acupressureonline.org

Information about the pressure points to treat arthritis

ADA Accessibility Guidelines for Buildings and Facilities

http://www.access-board.gov/adaag/html/adaag.htm

The latest guidelines, as amended through September 2002

American Academy of Medical Acupuncture

http://www.medicalacupuncture.org

Information on where to find a licensed acupuncturist

American Apitherapy Society

http://www.apitherapy.org

Information on bee sting therapy

American Association of Orthopaedic Medicine

http://www.aaomed.org

Provides information for patients on different treatment techniques and help with finding an orthopedic physician

American Chiropractic Association

http://www.acatoday.org

Provides information on the practice of chiropractic and where to find a licensed professional in your area

American College of Rheumatology

http://www.rheumatology.org

Provides news and resources for professionals as well as the general public on rheumatic conditions

American Osteopathic Association of Prolotherapy Integrative Pain Management

http://www.acopms.com

Comprehensive information on prolotherapy for health-care consumers

American Society for the Alexander Technique

http://www.alexandertech.org

Information about the Alexander Technique and where to find practitioners

American Volkssport Association

http://www.ava.org

Information about this walking club

American Yoga Association

http://www.americanyogaassociation.org

Information on yoga and where to find yoga practitioners

Arthritis Forum

http://forums.about.com/n/pfx/forum.aspx?nav=
messages&webtag=ab-arthritis

A fairly active online forum, mostly for rheumatoid arthritis

Arthritis Foundation

http://www.arthritis.org/chaptermap.php

Can help you find your local Arthritis Foundation chapter
office, which can assist you in finding support groups in
your area, as well as a wealth of information on national and
local programs for coping with arthritis, exercise programs,
the latest research, community events about arthritis, and
items that can help you live life to the fullest with arthritis.

Arthritis Foundation Self-Help Program

http://www.arthritis.org/self-help-program.php

Helps individuals learn the skills needed to build their own
self-management program so they can be active members
of their health-care team and handle the daily challenges
of the disease

Centers for Disease Control and Prevention

http://www.cdc.gov/arthritis/state_programs.htm

Information and a map where individuals can locate an
arthritis and other chronic disease program in their state

Feldenkrais Method of Somatic Education

http://www.feldenkrais.com

Provides information on the Feldenkrais Method and where to find teachers

International Association of Yoga Therapists

http://www.iayt.org

Information on yoga and where to find yoga practitioners

Lupus Research Institute

http://www.lupusresearchinstitute.org

Information on lupus, including advocacy and research

My RACentral

http://www.forums.healthcentral.com/discussion/rheumatoid-arthritis/forums

Online forum for people with rheumatoid arthritis

National Certification Commission for Acupuncture and Oriental Medicine

http://www.nccaom.org

Information on where to find a licensed acupuncturist

Walkablock Club of America

http://www.walkablock.com

Information about a walking club

Webwalking USA

http://walking.about.com/cs/measure/a/webwalkingusa
.htm

Information about a unique walking program

Yoga Alliance

http://www.yogaalliance.org

Information on yoga and where to find yoga practitioners

100-PLUS TYPES OF ARTHRITIS

Achilles tendinitis
Achondroplasia
Acromegalic arthropathy
Adhesive capsulitis
Adult onset Still's disease
Ankylosing spondylitis
Anserine bursitis
Arthritis of ulcerative colitis
Avascular necrosis
Behcet's syndrome
Bicipital tendinitis
Blount's disease
Brucellar spondylitis
Bursitis
Calcaneal bursitis
Calcium pyrophosphate dehydrate
Crystal deposition disease
Caplan's syndrome
Carpal tunnel syndrome
Chondrocalcinosis
Chondromalacia patellae
Chronic recurrent multifocal osteomyelitis
Chronic synovitis

Churg-Strauss syndrome
Cogan's syndrome
Corticosteroid-induced osteoporosis
Costosternal syndrome
CREST syndrome
Cryoglobulinemia
Degenerative joint disease
Dermatomyositis
Diabetic finger sclerosis
Diffuse idiopathic skeletal hyperostosis
Discitis
Discoid lupus erythematosus
Drug-induced lupus
Duchenne muscular dystrophy
Dupuytren's contracture
Ehlers-Danlos syndrome
Enteropathic arthritis
Epicondylitis
Erosive inflammatory osteoarthritis
Exercise-induced compartment syndrome
Fabry's disease
Familial Mediterranean fever
Farber's lipogranulomatosis
Felty's syndrome
Fibromyalgia
Fifth's disease
Flat feet
Foreign body synovitis
Freiberg's disease
Fungal arthritis
Gaucher's disease
Giant cell arteritis
Gonococcal arthritis
Goodpasture's syndrome
Gout

Granulomatous arteritis
Hemarthrosis
Hemochromatosis
Henoch-Schonlein purpura
Hepatitis B surface antigen disease
Hip dysplasia
Hurler syndrome
Hypermobility syndrome
Hypersensitivity vasculitis
Hypertrophic osteoarthropathy
Immune complex disease
Impingement syndrome
Jaccoud's arthropathy
Juvenile ankylosing spondylitis
Juvenile dermatomyositis
Juvenile rheumatoid arthritis
Kawasaki disease
Kienbock's disease
Legg-Calve-Perthes disease
Lesch-Nyhan syndrome
Linear scleroderma
Lipoid dermatoarthritis
Lofgren's syndrome
Lyme disease
Malignant synovioma
Marfan's syndrome
Medial plica syndrome
Metastatic carcinomatous arthritis
Mixed connective tissue disease
Mixed cryoglobulinemia
Mucopolysaccharidosis
Multicentric reticulohistiocytosis
Multiple epiphyseal dysplasia
Mycoplasmal arthritis
Myofascial pain syndrome

Neonatal lupus
Neuropathic arthropathy
Nodular panniculitis
Ochronosis
Olecranon bursitis
Osgood-Schlatter disease
Osteoarthritis
Osteochondromatosis
Osteogenesis imperfecta
Osteomalacia
Osteomyelitis
Osteonecrosis
Osteoporosis
Overlap syndrome
Pachydermoperiostosis Paget's disease
Palindromic rheumatism
Patellofemoral pain syndrome
Pellegrini-Stieda syndrome
Pigmented villonodular synovitis
Piriformis syndrome
Plantar fasciitis
Polyarteritis nodos
Polymyalgia rheumatic
Polymyositis
Popliteal cysts
Posterior tibial tendinitis
Pott's disease
Prepatellar bursitis
Prosthetic joint infection
Pseudoxanthoma elasticum
Psoriatic arthritis
Raynaud's phenomenon
Reactive arthritis/Reiter's syndrome
Reflex sympathetic dystrophy syndrome
Relapsing polychondritis

Retrocalcaneal bursitis
Rheumatic fever
Rheumatoid arthritis
Rheumatoid vasculitis
Rotator cuff tendinitis
Sacrolititis
Salmonella osteomyelitis
Sarcoidosis
Saturnine gout
Scheuermann's osteochondritis
Scleroderma
Septic arthritis
Seronegative arthritis
Shigella arthritis
Shoulder-hand syndrome
Sickle cell arthropathy
Sjogren's syndrome
Slipped capital femoral epiphysis
Spinal stenosis
Spondylolysis
Staphylococcus arthritis
Stickler syndrome
Subacute cutaneous lupus
Sweet's syndrome
Sydenham's chorea
Syphilitic arthritis
Systemic lupus erythematosus
Takayasu's arteritis
Tarsal tunnel syndrome
Tennis elbow
Tietze's syndrome
Transient osteoporosis
Traumatic arthritis
Trochanteric bursitis
Tuberculosis arthritis

Undifferentiated connective tissue syndrome
Urticarial vasculitis
Viral arthritis
Wegener's granulomatosis
Whipple's disease
Wilson's disease
Yersinia arthritis

NOTES

CHAPTER 1. ARTHRITIS: AN INTRODUCTION

American Academy of Orthopaedic Surgeons, Knee Osteoarthritis Statistics. http://orthoinfo.aaos.org/topic.cfm ?topic=A00399

L. Sharma et al., "Varus and Valgus Alignment and Incident and Progressive Knee Osteoarthritis," *Annals of Rheumatic Diseases* 69, no. 11 (November 2010): 1940–45.

CHAPTER 2. RHEUMATOID ARTHRITIS, GOUT, AND MORE

Arthritis Care & Rheumatism 58, no.1 (2008): 26–35.

Arthritis Care & Rheumatism 85, no. 1 (2008): 15–25.

M. A., Becker and G. E. Ruoff, "What Do I Need to Know About Gout?" *Journal of Family Practice* 59(6 suppl) (June 2010): S1–8.

Lupus Research Institute.

www.lupusresearchinstitute.org/.

CHAPTER 3. FINDING HEALTH-CARE PROFESSIONALS

www.consumerreports.org/health/doctors-hospitals/your
-doctor-relationship/how-to-choose-a-doctor/getting
-started/getting-started.htm.

American Academy of Orthopaedic Surgeons statistics:
www.beckersorthopedicandspine.com/lists-and-statis
tics/739-11-statistics-and-facts-about-orthopedics-and
-orthopedic-practices.

AAOS, "Orthopaedic Surgeon Shortage Predicted Due
to Soaring Joint Replacement Procedures," February 25,
2009, Las Vegas, NV, press release.

CHAPTER 4. GETTING A DIAGNOSIS

D. Aletaha et al., "2010 Rheumatoid Arthritis Classification Criteria: An American College of Rheumatology/Eu-
ropean League Against Rheumatism Collaborative
Initiative," *Arthritis & Rheumatism* 62, no. 9 (September
2010): 2569–81.

G. Madelin et al., "Sodium Inversion Recovery MRI of
the Knee Joint in Vivo at 7T," *Journal of Magnetic Resonance*, 207, no. 1 (November 2010): 42–52

CHAPTER 5. LET'S GET PHYSICAL: EXERCISE AND MOVEMENT THERAPY

M.F. Pisters et al., "Exercise Adherence Improving Long-Term Patient Outcome in Patients with Osteoarthritis of the Hip and/or Knee," *Arthritis Care & Research* 62, no. 8 (March 16, 2010):

CHAPTER 6. TREATING ARTHRITIS WITH MEDICATIONS

F. Clinard et al., "Association between Concomitant Use of Several Systemic NSAIDs and an Excess Risk of Adverse Drug Reaction," *European Journal of Clincal Pharmacology* 60, no. 4 (June 2004): 279–83.

Johns Hopkins: www.hopkins-arthritis.org/arthritis-info/rheumatoid-arthritis/rheum_treat.html.

S. Koelling and N. Miosge, "Sex Differences of Chondrogenic Progenitor Cells in Late Stages of Osteoarthritis," *Arthritis & Rheumatism* 62, no. 4 (April 2010): 1077–87.

Uloric Web site: www.uloric.com.

M. Whiteman et al., "Detection of Hydrogen Sulfide in Plasma and Knee-Joint Synovial Fluid from Rheumatoid Arthritis Patients: Relation to Clinical and Laboratory Measures of Inflammation, *Annals of the New York Academy of Sciences,* 1203 (August 17, 2010): 146–50.

CHAPTER 7. NUTRITIONAL, HERBAL, AND OTHER NATURAL SUPPLEMENTS

E. J. Blain et al., "*Boswellia frereana* (Frankincense) Suppresses Cytokine-Induced Matrix Metalloproteinase Expression and Production of Pro-inflammatory Molecules in Articular Cartilage," *Phytotherapy Research* 24, no. 6 (June 2010): 905–912.

M. Cameron et al., "Evidence of Effectiveness of Herbal Medicinal Products in the Treatment of Arthritis. Part I: Osteoarthritis," *Phytotherapy Research* 23, no. 11 (November 2009): 1497–515.

M. Cameron et al., "Evidence of Effectiveness of Herbal Medicinal Products in the Treatment of Arthritis: Part 2: Rheumatoid Arthritis," *Phytotherapy Research* 23, no. 12 (December 2009): 1647–62.

J. E. Chrubasik et al., "Evidence of effectiveness of herbal anti-inflammatory drugs in the treatment of painful osteoarthritis and chronic low back pain." *Phytotherapy Research* 21, no. 7, (July 2007): 675–83.

L. Deutsch, "Evaluation of the Effect of Neptune Krill Oil on Chronic Inflammation and Arthritic Symptoms," *Journal of the American College of Nutrition* 26, no. 1 (2007): 39–48.

E. Ernst, "Frankincense: Systematic Review," *British Medical Journal* 337 (December 17, 2008):a2813.

S-C Huang et al., "Vitamin B_6 Supplementation Improves Pro-inflammatory Responses in Patients with Rheumatoid

Arthritis, *European Journal of Clinical Nutrition* 64 (July 2010), online ahead of print.

M. Ierna et al., "Supplementation of Diet with Krill Oil Protects Against Experimental Rheumatoid Arthritis, *BMC Musculoskeletal Disorders* 11, no. 1 (June 29, 2010): 136.

N. Kimmatkar et al., "Efficacy and Tolerability of Boswellia Serrata Extract in Treatment of Osteoarthritis of Knee—a Randomized Double Blind Placebo Controlled Trial," *Phytomedicine* 10, no. 1 (January 2003): 3–7.

S.P. Myers et al., "A Combined Phase I and II Open Label Study on the Effects of a Seaweed Extract Nutrient Complex on Osteoarthritis," *Biologics* 4 (March 24, 2010): 33–44.

K. Pavelka et al. "Efficacy and Safety of Piascledine 300 versus Chondroitin Sulfate in a 6 Months Treatment Plus 2 Months Observation in Patients with Osteoarthritis of the Knee," *Clinical Rheumatology* 29, no. 6 (June 2010): 659–70.

R. Wall et al., "Fatty Acids from Fish: The Anti-inflammatory Potential of Long-Chain Omega-3 Fatty Acids," *Nutrition Reviews* 68, no. 5 (May 2010): 280–89.

Y. B. Yip and A. C. Tam, "An Experimental Study on the Effectiveness of Massage with Aromatic Ginger and Orange Essential Oil for Moderate-to-Severe Knee Pain Among the Elderly in Hong Kong," *Complementary Therapies in Medicine* 16, no. 3 (June 2008): 131–38.

CHAPTER 8. OTHER COMPLEMENTARY
AND ALTERNATIVE THERAPIES

L. Brosseau et al., "Low Level Laser Therapy for Osteo-arthritis and Rheumatoid Arthritis: A Metaanalysis," *Journal of Rheumatology* 27 (2000): 1961–69.

P. Efthimiou and M. Kukar, "Complementary and Alternative Medicine Use in Rheumatoid Arthritis: Proposed Mechanism of Action and Efficacy of Commonly Used Modalities," *Rheumatology International* 30, no. 5 (March 2010): 571–86.

G. Elkins et al., "Hypnotherapy for the Management of Chronic Pain," *International Journal of Clinical and Experimental Hypnosis* 55, no. 3 (July 2007): 275–87.

C. J. Herman et al., "Use of Complementary Therapies Among Primary Care Clinic Patients with Arthritis," *Preventing Chronic Diseases* 1, no. 4 (October 2004): A12.

S. R. Kim et al., "Critical Review of Prolotherapy for Osteoarthritis, Low Back Pain, and Other Musculoskeletal Conditions: A Physiatric Perspective," *American Journal of Physical Medicine Rehabilitation* 83, no. 5 (May 2004): 379–89.

M. A. Mont et al., "Pulsed Electrical Stimulation to Defer TKA in Patients with Knee Osteoarthritis," *Orthopedics* 29, no. 10 (October 2006): 887–92.

S. D. Ramsey et al., "Use of Alternative Therapies by Older Adults with Osteoarthritis," *Arthritis Care and Research* 45, no. 3 (June 2001): 222–27.

M. Suarez-Almazor et al., "A Randomized Controlled Trial of Acupuncture for Osteoarthritis of the Knee: Effects of Patient-Provider Communication," *Arthritis Care and Research* 62, no. 9 (September 2010): 1229–36.

A. J. Zautra et al., "Comparison of Cognitive Behavioral and Mindfulness Meditation Interventions on Adaptation to Rheumatoid Arthritis for Patients With and Without History of Recurrent Depression," *Journal of Consulting and Clinical Psychology* 76, no. 3 (June 2008): 408–21.

CHAPTER 9. SURGICAL OPTIONS

"Stem cell therapy may end joint replacement.": http://www.calgaryherald.com/health/Stem+cell+therapy+joint+replacement/3269020/story.html.

C.-C. Chang et al., "Anesthetic Management and Surgical Site Infections in Total Hip or Knee Replacement: A Population-Based Study," *Anesthesiology* 113, no. 2 (August 2010): 279–84.

CHAPTER 10. FOOD AND NUTRITION
FOR ARTHRITIS

I. Hafstrom I. et al., "A Vegan Diet Free of Gluten Improves the Signs and Symptoms of Rheumatoid Arthritis: The Effects on Arthritis Correlate with a Reduction in Antibodies to Food Antigens," *Rheumatology (Oxford)* 40, no. 10 (October 2001): 1175–79.

K. B. Hagen et al., "Dietary Interventions for Rheumatoid Arthritis," *Cochrane Database of Systematic Reviews*, no. 1 (January 21, 2009): CD006400.

K. K. Hanninen et al., "Antioxidants in Vegan Diet and Rheumatic Disorders," *Toxicology* 155, nos. 1–3 (November 30, 2000): 45–53.

S. Hurst et al., "Dietary Fatty Acids and Arthritis," *Prostaglandins, Leukotrienes and Essential Fatty Acids* 82, nos. 4–6 (April–June 2010): 315–18.

M. Hvatum et al., "The Gut-Joint Axis: Cross Reactive Food Antibodies in Rheumatoid Arthritis," *Gut* 55, no. 9 (September 2006): 1240–47.

J. McDougall et al., "Effects of a Very Low-Fat, Vegan Diet in Subjects with Rheumatoid Arthritis," *Journal of Alternative and Complementary Medicine* 8, no. 1 (February 2002): 71–75.

R. S. Panaush et al., "Diet Therapy for Rheumatoid Arthritis," *Arthritis and Rheumatism* 26 (1983): 462–71.

G. Smedslund et al., "Effectiveness and Safety of Dietary Interventions for Rheumatoid Arthritis: A Systematic Review of Randomized Controlled Trials," *Journal of the American Dietetic Association* 110, no. 5 (May 2010): 727–35.

CHAPTER 11. DAILY LIVING WITH ARTHRITIS

American College of Rheumatology, Pregnancy & Rheumatic Disease, April 5, 2007, http://www.rheumatology

.org/practice/clinical/patients/disease_and_conditions/
pregnancy.asp

B. Sleath et al., "Communication About Depression During Rheumatoid Arthritis Patient Visits," *Arthritis & Rheumatism* 59, no. 2 (February 15, 2008): 186–91.